# The 30 Day Heartburn Solution

## A 3-Step Nutrition Program to Stop Acid Reflux Without Drugs

By: Craig Fear, NTP

www.fearlesseating.net

Publishing services provided by 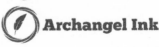 Archangel Ink

ISBN: 1942761627
ISBN-13: 978-1-942761-62-4

# DISCLAIMER

The information included in this book is for educational and informational purposes only and is not intended as a substitute for the medical advice of a licensed physician. I am not a medical doctor, and any advice I give is my opinion based on my own experience. As such, you should always seek the advice of your own health care professionals before acting upon anything I publish or recommend. By reading this book, you agree that my company and I are not responsible for your health or the health of your dependents. Use of the advice and other information contained in this book is at the sole choice and risk of the reader. Any statements or claims about the possible health benefits conferred by any foods or supplements have not been evaluated by the Food and Drug Administration and are therefore not intended to diagnose, treat, cure, or prevent any disease.

# Table of Contents

# Introduction

Several years ago, I gave a talk on digestive wellness at a local library. I was new to the area and was not expecting a big crowd, so I was pleasantly surprised when twenty-plus people showed up.

My talk focused on the acidity in the stomach. The reason, as you'll learn, is that proper acid secretion in the stomach dictates everything that happens further south in the digestive process. I explained in detail why heartburn is not caused by too much acid but, in fact, by NOT ENOUGH. I also explained the connection between the chronic use of heartburn medications and nutritional deficiencies, bone loss, and further digestive problems.

I figured much of the audience was on acid-reducing medications like TUMS and Rolaids or the more powerful acid-blockers like Nexium, Prilosec, and Zantac. After all, these are the most profitable drugs in America. Ads for them are all over the TV, radio, smartphones, and computer screens. Doctors give them out like candy. Hell, you don't even need a doctor anymore. A staggering variety of low-dose, over-the-counter versions of these meds are available everywhere. Standing in the digestive aide aisle of CVS is now like standing in the cereal aisle of your supermarket.

I also figured that those taking these medications were doing so under the mistaken belief that their stomach was producing TOO MUCH acid. Besides the media and their doctors, there's an even more important influence that drives this belief—their symptoms. After all, if there's a burning sensation in the chest region, it's logical to think that there's too much acid.

I thought there would be at least a few who questioned me on this poorly understood, unpublicized, and much-less-profitable theory of heartburn. I was prepared to explain that this was not a theory I personally came up with. I was prepared to say that the practice of boosting the acidity in the stomach to prevent acidity in the esophagus was actually being used by thousands of other doctors and alternative healers all around the country, and that I was having great success myself using it with clients. I was prepared to share my resources for those who wanted to explore further.

But no one debated me on it. At the end of my talk, people even applauded. I was shocked. I guess that's because with a little education it's not that hard to understand. However, not everyone was as convinced as I'd thought.

A few days later, I got an email from Sarah, one of the attendees. A long-time heartburn sufferer, she was intrigued by my talk. She went to her doctor, who was prescribing her Nexium, an acid-blocking medication, and told him about my talk and the competing theory that heartburn is a result of low acid production. Not surprisingly, the doctor convinced her I was dead wrong and that all the research and science supports the overproduction of acid as the root cause of heartburn.

Boy, did she let me have it in her email. In a somewhat demeaning tone, she told me that I'm not a doctor, that I should do further research, and that the theory of low acid is flat-out wrong.

I didn't take the email personally. After all, many health issues today are hot-button topics, and they can trigger sensitive emotions in people. Just take a look at the comments in health-related articles and blog posts these days. It's craaaaaazy! My blog, *Fearless Eating*, gets its fair share of sarcasm, anger, and insults. You'd better have some thick skin to write a nutrition blog today. But I was helping too many people and was too confident in the science that supports the under-production of acid as the root cause of heartburn to be dissuaded. In a few days, I'd forgotten about it entirely.

Two YEARS later, I received an email with the subject line that read, "I owe you an apology."

It was from Sarah.

She wrote:

*"I attended a lecture you gave at the Forbes Library a few years or so ago on the subject of acid reflux and heartburn. I was intrigued, but when I checked with my gastroenterologist, he assured me that the science supported his approach, and so I wrote you suggesting you limit yourself to the science.*

*Meanwhile, I got worse and worse and found myself enduring heartburn even though I was taking 40 mg of Nexium daily. I reconsidered, if not the science, at least the logic of your assertions. If my stomach had virtually no acid as a result of taking Nexium, how could I be suffering from hyperacidity (too much acid)? So I decided to try some science on myself, to test the hypothesis that hypoacidity (low acid) was the problem. While actually suffering heartburn and contemplating taking a second Nexium of the day, I took acid instead. Well, it worked, and I continued my experimentation.*

*I have to say, I was skeptical of the 'caused by not enough acid' theory, but now I am convinced. I feel like an addict cured."*

Let me be clear on that last sentence. This book is not a miracle cure. People look for cures these days, and I agree that medicine holds that potential for many. Modern science has made remarkable advances in treatments for so many conditions. But too many of us wait for cures, failing to realize a simple change in diet and lifestyle can do so much for our health. Heartburn is a perfect example. It doesn't develop overnight. No one contracts heartburn like malaria or the HIV virus. There is nothing magical about stopping heartburn. As you'll see, it's a simple matter of cause and effect. Stop the cause and the effect will cease. Call it a cure if you want. I just call it a commonsense solution.

Nor is the crux of this book about supplementation. Sarah helped herself by taking some acid, a very common approach in the holistic health world and one that I will explore and explain. But often, in fact, supplementation isn't even needed. Dietary changes are usually all it takes.

Thus, a strong emphasis will be put on nutrition and diet. But I'm not talking about the conventional dietary advice you've probably heard a thousand times over. You know, eliminate triggers, reduce stress, stop overeating, and reduce fat. Though this may help, it is unfortunately *extremely limiting*. For starters, it tells you nothing about *what you should eat*, only what you shouldn't. And what you should eat is much more important for stopping heartburn than what you shouldn't eat.

This book is divided into four parts. Part I will explain the science of heartburn as simply as possible. By using a few simple analogies, I'll help you understand how digestion works in a nutshell, why heartburn manifests, and why heartburn is often related to so many other digestive problems.

You see, it's rare that I see someone for just heartburn. There's usually other complaints as well—bloating, inflammation, fatigue, weight gain, nausea, constipation, gallbladder problems, and irritable bowel syndrome (IBS), to name a few.

By understanding digestion in its totality, we can better understand why heartburn causes so many other problems and why reducing the acidity in the stomach through acid-reducing medications exacerbates those problems. In the process, you may experience relief from your other digestive symptoms, as well. In fact, I would expect it.

Part II will explore the foundation for the 3-Step Plan, which are dietary changes. Nutrition has become as controversial as politics and religion these days, so Part II will clear up that confusion and detail what I call "the five pillars of real food" that we'll be using in the 3-Step Plan.

Part III will outline the 3-Step Plan in detail. Using Part II as the foundation, you'll see this plan is not only designed to stop heartburn, it's also designed to *make you healthy*. Acid-reducing meds can do the former as well but not the latter.

And Part IV will include recipes and meal ideas for helping you put the 3-Step Plan into action.

My goal in this book is very simple. I want you to overcome your heartburn fast—REALLY fast. Like Sarah, there's a good chance your heartburn will stop well before 30 days pass. I have seen people with decades of heartburn turn their symptoms around within a matter of days. I have seen others where it takes more time. Everyone is different, and some respond quicker than others. Regardless, if you follow the 3-Step Plan, I am confident that your symptoms will improve dramatically in 30 days. More important, you'll create a foundation for a heartburn-free, healthy life well beyond that.

# Part I

Understanding Heartburn

# 1

# What Are Heartburn and GERD?

## What is Heartburn?

Our stomach produces hydrochloric acid (HCl) to help us break down and digest our food. Under normal conditions, we don't feel this acid because our stomach also produces a protective mucosal barrier between the acid and our stomach lining. Heartburn occurs when acid from your stomach refluxes back into your esophagus. Thus, heartburn is often referred to as "acid reflux." Unlike the stomach, your esophagus does not have a mucosal lining to protect itself from stomach acid. This acid burns the lining of your esophagus, which lies just in front of the heart, and thus we experience heartburn.

When this happens occasionally, it's really no big deal. Just like with a minor cut on your skin, your esophagus has the ability to repair itself pretty quickly. All of us, at one time or another, have probably experienced the sensation of heartburn.

But heartburn becomes a problem when it starts to happen on more than rare occasions.

## What is Gastro-Esophageal Reflux Disease (GERD)?

GERD is chronic heartburn. Chronic means it occurs at least a few times per week. Over time, chronic heartburn can erode the lining of the esophagus and cause a whole host of problems. While heartburn is the main symptom of GERD, sometimes people are diagnosed with GERD without heartburn. Other symptoms manifest such as coughing, asthma-like symptoms, difficulty swallowing, a hoarse voice, continually clearing one's throat, and a sour taste in one's mouth.

In 2004, 64.6 million medications were prescribed by doctors for GERD, accounting for over half of all prescriptions for digestive disorders.[1] That *does* *not* include over-the-counter medications, which don't need a doctor's prescription.

GERD is usually diagnosed through its main symptom, heartburn. Sometimes an upper endoscopy, a procedure in which a tube is swallowed into the upper gastrointestinal tract, can confirm GERD as well. A miniature camera can detect the scarring in the esophagus.

However, GERD can occur even without the visual evidence. Still, when this is observed, it's a sign that the chronic reflux of acid is becoming dangerous.

GERD can lead to another condition called Barrett's esophagus, which manifests when the lining of the esophagus becomes permanently damaged through chronic exposure to stomach acid. There are no known drugs or even natural therapies that can reverse it. This permanent scarring can lead to esophageal cancer. Though Barrett's esophagus is still somewhat rare, heartburn and GERD are not.

## Why are so Many People Experiencing Heartburn and GERD?

To best answer this question, I'll start with a more important question that I think can help us answer this question more effectively.

That question is, **"Why are so many people experiencing digestive disorders today?"**

I ask that question because, as we'll see, heartburn and GERD set up a domino-like effect of other digestive problems. As I explained in the introduction, it is relatively rare that anyone comes to see me for just heartburn. There are usually a variety of other connected problems such as bloating, gas, dysbiosis, diarrhea, constipation, gallbladder problems, intestinal pain, and more clinically defined digestive illnesses such as IBS, Crohn's disease, and ulcerative colitis, the rates of which are escalating everywhere, including in our children.

According to the United States Department of Health and Human Services, 70 million Americans experience digestive disorders at a cost of over 140 **billion** dollars per year.[2]

By understanding why and how heartburn and GERD manifest, we can understand why and how so many other digestive problems manifest, as well. In so doing, we can not only set the stage for overcoming heartburn and GERD, but in the process, build a foundation for good long-term digestive health and overall health.

And this is **exactly** the problem with conventional treatments. They can free you of acid refluxing into your esophagus, but they often do so **at the expense of your long-term health**. They fix one problem but in the process cause a multitude of other ones for which more drugs are often prescribed.

My 3-Step Plan will stop the burning in your chest, *and* it also holds the potential to improve other associated health problems.

To understand this clearly, let's start by taking a brief tour of the digestive tract. And let's keep it as simple as possible. I will use three analogies to explain how each of the three parts of the digestive system—the upper GI (Gastrointestinal), the middle GI, and the lower GI—works, because when you understand how things are supposed to work, you can then understand how easy it is for things to go wrong. And then you'll see how easy it can be to turn things around via natural means.

# 2

# The Blender, the Sponge, and the Rainforest

The most important thing to understand is that digestion is a north to south process. It flows like a river. It begins upstream in the brain, mouth, and stomach and ends downstream in the large intestine. And just like a river, what happens upstream influences what happens downstream. We have all sorts of drugs, medications, and high-tech procedures that treat digestive problems where they occur downstream, but so often, the root of the problem lies upstream. And upstream is exactly where heartburn occurs.

## The Blender

Your upper GI tract consists of your mouth, esophagus, stomach, gallbladder, and pancreas. Their job is akin to a blender.

Digestion actually starts in your brain with the thought of food, which makes you salivate. When you chew, you mechanically start breaking down the food, and you also salivate. Saliva contains enzymes that start to chemically break down the food. When you swallow, food travels through your esophagus to your stomach. So far so good, right?

The stomach is where things start to heat up, literally and figuratively. The most basic role of your stomach is to blend your food. It does this primarily through the action of pepsin and hydrochloric acid (HCl). Pepsin is a digestive enzyme that breaks down protein. It requires HCl and thus a highly acid environment to function. Your stomach contains millions of hydrochloric acid-producing cells. HCl and pepsin break down your food just like a blender. HCl also helps to disinfect our food and kill any potential pathogens such as harmful bacteria and viruses.

We need HCl, and we need its production to be *strong*. Strong HCl production is like having the speed of the blender on high. That's good! HCl is so strong, in fact, that if you removed some of it from your stomach, it would burn a hole in your shirt. But again, we don't feel it because we have a mucosal lining in our stomach that protects us from it.

When food leaves the stomach, it enters the duodenum, the upper part of the small intestine. Proper acid production signals the pancreas to release bicarbonate, a baking soda-like solution that deacidifies the acid so that the next phase of digestion can occur. The pancreas then adds in further digestive enzymes, and the gallbladder adds bile. You know those manual "pulse" settings on a blender that you use when things are mostly blended but not quite 100%? That's how I look at the role of the gallbladder and pancreas. They add some additional pulses on the blender so that by the time our food leaves our upper GI, almost everything is thoroughly digested.

Now your food is like the consistency of a creamy soup. Kinda gross, I know, but that's a good thing. This sets the stage for easy absorption in the small intestines.

## The Sponge

Now food is ready to enter the middle part of the GI tract, the small intestines. Imagine your small intestines like a long, hollow tube, and the walls of the tube are made out of a sponge.

The primary role of the small intestines is to absorb the nutrients in your food. This happens easily when the food has been broken down into its component parts by your upper GI, meaning that fats are broken down into fatty acids, proteins are broken down into amino acids, and carbohydrates are broken down into simple sugars. These nutrients move through the intestinal wall like water moves through a sponge. The tiny little holes in a sponge allow water to move through, but not bigger particles. So the nutrients move through the sponge while those larger particles that should not move through, like fiber and other waste materials, move into your large intestines.

The nutrients that move through the intestinal wall are carried by your bloodstream to all the tissues of your body for nourishment and energy.

Pretty simple, right?

## The Amazon Rainforest

Now the food, which is becoming less soup-like and more poop-like (yeah, I made that one up all by myself), moves into the lower GI, the large intestine. The analogy I like to use here is that the large intestine is to the body what the Amazon rainforest is to planet Earth. The Amazon rainforest is the most fertile region on our planet, teeming with millions of different life forms. This vast and rich diversity of life plays vital roles in keeping the rest of our planet healthy.

So too the large intestine is the most fertile region in your body. It is teeming with life in the form of trillions upon trillions of microscopic bacteria. And that's a good thing because we could not live without them. In fact, there are so many bacteria that live in us (and on us) that there are actually ten times more of them than cells in our body. Crazy, huh? About five hundred different species of bacteria have been identified so far.

As unpleasant as it may be to think that trillions of microscopic little buggers are crawling around in you, they are absolutely *essential* to your health and survival. Here are just a few roles they play:

- Manufacture B vitamins and vitamin K.
- Produce butyric acid, which keeps the bowel wall healthy.
- Break down toxins.
- Prevent infection by other microbes.
- Promote immune system health.

- Promote hormonal health.
- Regulate bowel movements.
- Improve mineral absorption.

And that's just the tip of the iceberg. In fact, many consider these bacteria and the roles they play a new frontier of science. Researchers are learning more and more about them all the time. But we do know that when these bacteria are healthy and thriving so too do we thrive just as our planet thrives through the richness and diversity of different life forms. Destroy the diversity of life and serious consequences develop. I'm sure you can see where I'm going with this. But under normal circumstances, once the bacteria finish their job, whatever waste material is left over, we excrete.

So that's how digestion is supposed to work in a nutshell. That is, of course, a very simplistic explanation, but it serves our purpose well enough. Now let's go through it again and see what happens when things go wrong and why the acidity in our stomach is so important.

# 3

# When the Blender Slows Down

So the first thing that goes wrong is the easiest to understand. We eat on the go. We eat mindlessly in front of our computers and TVs. We eat when we're stressed. Simply put, we don't relax, and we don't chew thoroughly. So right away, we're assaulting our stomach with food that has not been properly salivated or thoroughly chewed. Now the stomach has some extra work to do.

But worse than that are the things that can compromise the production of hydrochloric acid, leading to a state known as hypochlorhydria. Hypochlorhydria simply means low stomach acid production. Remember, HCl is akin to a blender. What happens if that blender slows down? In other words, what happens when our HCl does not get produced properly? Food doesn't digest as well. So the million-dollar question is…

**What Causes Low Stomach Acid?**

There are two main factors to consider.

**1. Age**

Some practitioners believe age is the primary influence. After all, HCl declines with age,[1] just like your hormones, your muscle mass, your hearing, your memory, and pretty much everything else. But here's the thing: the incidence of heartburn *increases* with age.[2] This is fairly common knowledge. If we are to believe that heartburn is caused by too much acid, then why don't younger people experience more heartburn than older people?

While age is clearly an influence, I don't believe it's the primary cause. Just because we get older doesn't mean we should experience heartburn and GERD. A 1996 study in the *Journal of Gastroenterology and Hepatology* found that elderly people don't automatically experience decline in digestive function but rather are more susceptible to it due to natural aging factors.[3] So then what are the factors that make us more susceptible to heartburn as we age? Truth be told, I do believe age is the main factor, but a different sort of age: our modern age.

## 2. Diet and stress

Chronic diseases are escalating in industrialized societies. This is not hard to see. It is a rare person today who does not know a friend or family member affected by cancer or heart disease. Autoimmune issues are skyrocketing. Obesity and type 2 diabetes are off the charts. The four A's in kids—autism, ADHD, allergies, and asthma—-are also on the rise. Each generation today seems to get sicker and sicker at younger and younger ages.

While there are many forces responsible for this, I believe our modern diet and lifestyle are the biggest culprits. After all, poor diet and lifestyle choices deplete the body of nutrients. And I believe this is the true underlying reason for compromised acidity in the stomach. We will take a lot closer look at diet in the next chapter. As you'll see, even health-conscious people today are not getting the nutrients they need for overall good health.

Stress is another factor, and it's interesting to consider because it's often blamed for the *overproduction* of acid. Many people report that their heartburn symptoms increase during times of high stress. Reducing your stress is part of the conventional treatment recommendations for heartburn. Doctors will tell you to control your stress and of course will give you an antacid at the same time. But let's look a little closer at stress to understand why it may contribute to low stomach acid.

There are two branches to our autonomic nervous system, which is the part of our nervous system that works involuntarily, meaning we don't control its function. The two branches are the parasympathetic and the sympathetic, and they work in opposition to each other, meaning when one is active the other is at rest and vice versa. Our parasympathetic system is responsible for bodily activities that require a state of rest. Our sympathetic system is responsible for the stress response also known as the fight-or-flight response. **Digestion is a parasympathetic activity.** We need to be in a restful state for good digestion, as a restful state will bring more blood and oxygen to the internal organs. The stress response signals the body to do the opposite and thus to bring blood and oxygen to our muscles. We breathe harder and our heart pumps harder. It is primarily a survival mechanism that makes us either run from an emergency situation or fight one.

It stands to reason that acid production may not be optimal during times of stress. In fact, research confirms that stress has a wide range of both short- and long-term negative effects on gastric function and can lead to an assortment of digestive problems *including* heartburn and GERD.[4,5]

Furthermore, the sympathetic nervous system is meant to be activated only *on occasion*. Of course, modern life is *so stressful* that many people today live in a perpetual state of stress. We all know people like that in our lives. The classic type-A personality would be a good example.

**We know that chronic stress degrades the functioning of every system in our body.** Cortisol, the primary stress hormone, shuts off the production of other metabolic pathways. Digestion, hormone production, and mental function, to name a few, are not priorities for the body in times of stress. When we are stressed all the time, we become depleted, tired, and worn out. We come home exhausted and hungry, and we overeat or drink too much to numb away the stress. We wake up exhausted and need caffeine and sugar to get us through the day. Through the years, our digestion weakens.

Now let's ask the next million-dollar question…

**What happens when we have low stomach acid?**

Let's answer that question in a roundabout way by asking another question first.

What forms the foundation of the Standard American Diet (SAD)?

Essentially, sugar and refined carbohydrates.

Think of the standard American breakfast—sugary cereal, fruit juices, muffins, bagels, pastries, sugary pancakes, donuts, sugary coffee drinks, etc. Pasta, bread, cookies, cakes, ice cream, chocolate, candy, and sweetened drinks like soda and sports drinks form a major part of the rest of the day's meals and snacks.

And as you'll see in the next chapter, the standard low-fat dietary advice put forth by doctors and dietitians is exacerbating the overconsumption of these foods. The junk food industry is happy to oblige with a dizzying array of poor-quality food that is absolutely loaded with sugar but is slapped with a low-fat label.

Now remember, our stomach is a warm, moist environment. It's almost 100 degrees in there. Fermentation, the process by which sugars get broken down, produces gas as a byproduct. Fermentation likes warmth as it happens more quickly and more efficiently in its presence. If you've ever fermented vegetables, you know they ferment more quickly in the summer than in the winter.

In the presence of low stomach acid, the sugars in carbohydrates can ferment and lead to the production of excess gas. Bloating, belching, and bad breath are some of the symptoms that result. The maldigested mass of food and the gas that results builds up in the stomach and can start to put pressure on the lower esophageal sphincter (LES), the valve that keeps the stomach separate from the esophagus. Over time, the LES can weaken through this continuous increased pressure.[6]

As pressure builds, some of the acidic contents of the stomach can reflux back into the esophagus. And as we've seen, unlike the stomach, the lining of the esophagus is not meant for acid, so it burns. As previously described, this burning of the lining of the esophagus is known as heartburn. ***So the root cause of heartburn is the under-production of stomach acid.*** This sounds counterintuitive because we've been so thoroughly conditioned to believe the *complete opposite,* which sounds logical. Certainly if we experience a burning sensation, it makes sense to think there is an excess of acid. And certainly, Big Pharma loves to keep both the public and doctors thinking this way. Yes, the primary reason doctors believe heartburn is caused by too much acid is due to the heavy influence from the pharmaceutical industry. Unfortunately, doctors get much of their information from drug representatives, industry-sponsored conferences, and industry-funded research in medical journals.

# 4

# The Problem with Heartburn Medications

Heartburn medications can be divided into two types, acid-neutralizers and acid-blockers. Acid-neutralizers, also known as antacids, are low-tech versions such as TUMS and Rolaids, and they alkalinize the stomach for a brief period. There are two types of acid-blockers: histamine H2 blockers and proton pump inhibitors (PPIs). H2 blockers like Zantac and Pepcid interfere with a chemical pathway that signals the stomach to produce acid. PPIs such as Nexium, Prilosec, and Prevacid are even more powerful. They work by directly shutting down the acid-producing cells in the stomach.

Both acid-neutralizers and acid-blockers compromise the acidity in the stomach **ON PURPOSE**. In doing so, they relieve the burning sensation of heartburn. So I'm not denying that they work. However, by altering the naturally acidic environment in the stomach, they cause a whole host of other problems in the digestive process.

Remember, the stomach is **supposed to be highly acidic**. Taking acid-suppressing medications is akin to reducing the blender speed of the stomach, which causes all the problems discussed above in the digestive process. So while antacids and acid-blockers help relieve the burning sensation of heartburn, they do not address the underlying cause, which is TOO LITTLE acid in the stomach. Thus they perpetuate the vicious cycle of chronic digestive problems including, of course, the very conditions they are designed to treat, namely heartburn and GERD. This is why most people who take these drugs have to continually take them. If they stop, the heartburn comes right back. The irony in this is just unbelievable. See why acid-blocking medications are the most profitable drugs in America?

Now let's take a look at how lowering your stomach acid production can cause further problems in each of the three phases of our digestive tract.

## Overgrowth of Bacteria in the Stomach

Though the bacteria in our digestive system are heavily concentrated in our intestines, there are some that can survive our stomach's acidity and take up residence there. One in particular, *Helicobacter pylori* (*H. pylori*), poses an interesting problem.

*H. pylori* lives naturally in our stomach but is not problematic if our acid production is strong. Remember, stomach acid plays a dual role of not only breaking down our food but also purifying it. Strong acid production kills parasites, yeasts, and viruses but also keeps *H. pylori* in check. So though it can survive in the presence of strong acid, it can't thrive. However, low stomach acid production presents an opportunity for *H. pylori*.

For decades, gastritis (inflammation in the stomach lining) and stomach ulcers were attributed to stress and the overproduction of stomach acid. It wasn't until recently that research found the true cause of ulcers is the overgrowth of *H. pylori*. *H. pylori* is able to burrow into the lining of the stomach and compromise the mucosal barrier that separates the lining from stomach acid. But it can only do this when the acidity in our stomach becomes compromised. A vicious cycle then develops in which *H. pylori* further inhibits stomach acid secretion.[1]

Ironically, one of the best treatments to eradicate *H. pylori* is to use an antibiotic in combination with Prilosec. Prilosec lowers the acidity to the point where the antibiotic can kill *H. pylori*. It has made more archaic and risky surgical treatments for ulcers null and void.[2]

However, acid-suppressing drugs increase the risk of future *H. pylori* infection, because *H. pylori* can only establish itself in a stomach environment that is acid-compromised. The antibiotic may kill the *H. pylori*, but the antacid medication is further compromising stomach acidity. This sets the stage for another vicious cycle as low stomach acid results in heartburn and GERD.

Yikes!

## When the Sponge Gets Leaky

Moving further south, this compromised acidity can impact the ability of the pancreas and gallbladder to do their jobs as well. Proper acid production in the stomach signals the pancreas to release digestive enzymes and the gallbladder to release bile. Without strong acidity, the pancreas and gallbladder don't get the proper signals.

Food that does not get broken down properly also sets the stage for bacterial overgrowth in the lower intestines. We experience further bloating and gas, which can lead to a further buildup of pressure in the stomach.

So beyond just heartburn, when this happens on a regular basis, all sorts of chronic intestinal problems ensue as well. Now we have the development of all these conditions that end in "itis." Conditions that end in "itis" refer to issues of inflammation. So now we have ileitis (inflammation of the ileum), colitis, diverticulitis, ulcerative colitis, and Crohn's disease. Many believe this small intestinal bacterial overgrowth sets the stage for IBS, a condition that's becoming more commonly diagnosed when patients exhibit chronic abdominal pain, bloating, and, often, alternating diarrhea and constipation. Doctors have no answers for IBS.

Furthermore, the maldigested food can start to compromise the lining of the small intestine, setting up a condition known as increased intestinal permeability or leaky gut. In our sponge analogy, imagine that the spongy wall becomes a lot less spongy.

The tiny little holes that are supposed to only allow the smallest nutrients through now start allowing large particles through.

When this happens, the immune system becomes activated. Seventy percent of our immune system resides in our gut. When undigested particles start passing through, food allergies and sensitivities can develop. This sets the stage for a whole host of immune issues such as asthma, skin conditions, parasitic and viral infections, and even autoimmune conditions.

## When the Rainforest Loses Its Diversity

OK, let's keep going south. Now this maldigested food assaults the large intestine. Keep in mind that of the trillions of bacteria that reside in our large intestine, about 85% of them are beneficial and about 15% are pathogenic. In a healthy gut, those 85% keep the 15% in check. Thus, the 15% don't harm us. But in an unhealthy gut, those 15% can start to proliferate. In particular, they will feed on too many sugars and carbohydrates in the diet. As we've seen, too many sugars and carbs is the foundation of the very unhealthy Standard American Diet.

But worse than that is our epidemic overuse of antibiotics. Antibiotics, which translates as "anti-life," are prescribed by doctors to kill harmful bacteria within us. While this may be necessary, antibiotics do not discriminate between good and bad bacteria and in the process of killing the bad ones also kill the good ones. Today it is not uncommon for people to take antibiotics on multiple occasions for months at a time. This can compromise the diversity of beneficial bacteria and may have far-reaching health consequences. It's akin to the destruction of the Amazon rainforest and its effect on the rest of our planet. The long-term implications may be dire if we don't stop.

## Why the Conventional "Natural" Approach Rarely Works

Of course, not everyone who experiences heartburn and GERD takes medications. Many doctors are aware of the long-term problems with acid-blockers and encourage their patients to manage their symptoms through diet and lifestyle changes. Unfortunately, much of what passes for diet and lifestyle changes in the medical profession is extremely limiting. Perhaps you've tried some of these more conventional "natural" approaches and perhaps it's why you're reading this book, because chances are, while it may have helped a little, it didn't completely stop your heartburn.

The conventional natural medical approach to heartburn can be summed up in four statements:

1. Avoid your triggers. These differ for everyone but the common ones are chocolate, coffee, garlic, onions, tomatoes, citrus, alcohol, and spicy foods.
2. Don't overeat.
3. Limit your stress.
4. Limit your intake of fat.

Do a Google search, and website after website after website will tell you some minor variation of that. Losing weight (though they don't tell you how) and stopping smoking (not exactly easy if you're addicted) are some of the other common suggestions.

Avoiding your triggers is good advice. Obviously, if something exacerbates your heartburn, don't eat it. But doing so won't solve the underlying issue. With my 3-Step Plan, we're looking to restore the acidity in the stomach and bolster the integrity of the GI lining so that down the line, unless you're truly allergic to those foods, you should be able to consume them again in moderation.

Not overeating and limiting your stress are also good advice. But that's a lot easier said than done, isn't it? I'm here to tell you that not overeating will be A LOT easier on my 3-Step Plan. And one of the reasons is that we absolutely will not be following the advice to limit your intake of fat, which is often misrepresented as eating too many calories or, you know, just overeating. In fact, a 1998 study in the journal *Gut* found that fatty foods *do not* influence heartburn when calories are not overconsumed.[3]

The study compared a group of healthy subjects to a group of patients with GERD. They fed both groups a high-fat meal and then a balanced-fat meal of equal calories. In both cases, "the high-fat meal did not increase the rate of reflux episodes nor exposure to esophageal acid in either group regardless of body posture."

As we'll learn, not eating fat is *very stressful* to the body. It also sets the stage for cravings and the overconsumption of sugar and carbohydrates. Furthermore, healthy fats have anti-inflammatory properties that will help heal the gastric lining.

But that's just the tip of the iceberg. To truly restore proper stomach function and stop heartburn once and for all, we need to take a much different approach.

And that's where real food comes in.

# Part II

Understanding Real Food

# 5

# Weston Price and the Five Real Food Pillars

In my practice, I offer a free 30-minute consult to all potential clients. This initial session allows me to see if I can help someone first before they commit to working with me. It also allows me to explain how I work with folks so the client can understand what's involved. I frequently say that one of the ways in which my approach differs from others in the nutrition field is that I work with real food.

The reaction I get is almost universal. Quiet head nods.

It sounds good, right? I mean how could anyone possibly disagree with eating real food? But if I were to ask those people what they think real food means, the majority would say something to the effect of, "Eat more fruits, vegetables, and whole grains, and cut down on fats, especially red meat."

And when I question them about their current diet, I'm given a long list of foods that masquerade as real food such as low-fat milk, low-fat yogurt, soy milk, breakfast cereals, processed fruit juices, imitation butter spreads like Smart Balance, imitation egg products like Egg Beaters, and a whole slew of fake, soy-based imitation meat products.

I call this the Health-Conscious Standard American Diet. And though it may be slightly less unhealthy than the Standard

American Diet, it's still a low-fat diet based on a lot of refined foods and refined carbohydrates. Breads, muffins, boxed cereals, pastries, pasta, and rice are the everyday staples. Animal proteins are usually lean proteins such as boneless chicken breasts and white fish fillets trimmed of fat and skin. All dairy products are low in fat or completely devoid of it. The use of highly processed, poor-quality, polyunsaturated vegetable oils is almost universal, especially canola and soybean oils.

Many of these clients are also struggling with sugar cravings. Further questioning reveals uncontrollable cravings for sugar in all its myriad forms such as sweetened coffee drinks, ice cream, candy, cakes, cookies, and chocolate.

With some education, I help these people start to understand why what they think is real food is not really real food. And this is so important for heartburn as well! Because understanding real food is key to not only managing your heartburn but to *stopping it once and for all.*

## The Lessons of Dr. Weston Price

The best way I've learned to explain real food without getting bogged down in the controversial world of nutritional science is to explain the research of Dr. Weston A. Price.

Dr. Price was a prominent dentist in his day and was head of the research division of the American Dental Association from 1914-1928.

Dr. Price was part of a rising tide of scientists and researchers concerned about the rapidly changing food supply in the early decades of the twentieth century. Heavily processed foods such as canned goods, refined grains, and refined sugars, which Dr. Price called the "foods of commerce," were becoming more common. The supermarket was in the early stages of supplanting the backyard garden and the family farm as America's primary food source.

In these early decades, Dr. Price was seeing a dramatic rise in the incidence of dental problems, including cavities, root canals, deformed dental arches, and crooked teeth, especially in children. He was also seeing a strong correlation between dental problems and other physical problems, and he suspected the foods of commerce were at the root of these growing trends.

Dr. Price decided to investigate. His investigation and research took him far beyond the world of universities, laboratories, textbooks, and statistics. In the 1930s, Dr. Price traveled to all corners of the world and sought out the most isolated cultures he could find at a time when there were still cultures untouched by modern civilization.

He lived with and studied the Inuit in Alaska, Native Americans in the Florida Everglades, African tribes, the Maori of New Zealand, the Aboriginals of Australia, Swiss villagers in remote regions of the Alps, Gaelic populations of the Hebrides Islands off the coast of Scotland, and South American Indians.

He summarized his findings in his book *Nutrition and Physical Degeneration,* which was first published in 1939.

## An Interesting Question

Have you ever wondered what cultures did before the advent of modern dentistry? It's an interesting question, isn't it? Today we take for granted that we need to get our teeth cleaned, cavities filled, wisdom teeth pulled, and have a bunch of metal awkwardly glued to our teeth for a few years as teenagers. It's almost crazy to think of life without dentists today.

Well, unbelievable as it may sound, Dr. Price found absolutely no need for modern dentistry in any of the cultures he studied. Besides incredibly low rates of cavities, he also found almost no evidence of further dental problems such as crowded and crooked teeth. I know that's hard to imagine in this day and age when there's not just one but five, ten, maybe even a few dozen dentists in every town and city in America.

## The Diet Connection

Dr. Price also studied the diets of these cultures. He studied not only what they were eating but *why* they were eating it and the techniques they used to prepare it. He made the connection between their excellent dental health and their native foods. Let's briefly examine three aspects of their diets that differ greatly from our modern diets.

## 1. No processed foods

Obviously, Dr. Price found no processed foods. This of course included refined sugars and refined carbohydrates, the two mainstays of most modern diets. Refined foods are stripped of their nutrients and do not supply the body with the building blocks for good health. These cultures' remote locations kept them removed from the transportation systems necessary to deliver the foods of commerce. That was about to change in the coming decades as the forces of industrialization would creep into almost every corner of our world.

## 2. Animals were raised on pasture

Secondly, these cultures had an intimate understanding of the connection between the health of their animals and their own health. Domesticated animals like cows, sheep, lamb, chickens, and goats were all raised on pasture. They ate what nature intended them to eat, namely grass, leaves, shrubs, and, in the case of chickens, some insects and bugs as well.

The modern method of raising animals, the factory farm, confines animals in small spaces so they can be injected with growth hormones and fed grains, soybeans, and other unnatural industrial byproducts to fatten them faster and cheaper than if they were on pasture. This makes them sick, for which they're regularly given antibiotics. It also makes them deficient in nutrients.

Dr. Price took samples of each culture's food and sent them back to the US for laboratory analysis. On average, he found the diets of these cultures were ***TEN times higher in vitamins A, D, E, and K.***

## 3. Soil integrity was maintained

Thirdly, these cultures had a great understanding and respect for their soil. They knew how to maintain the complexity and vitality of their soil to ensure the future health of their food supply. Modern practices, including monoculture and the use of chemicals, are withdrawing nutrients from the soil faster than they can be replaced. As a result, Dr. Price found the diets of these cultures were **FOUR times higher in minerals.** And this was back in the 1930s.

In short, none of these cultures were eating anything resembling the food in our modern-day supermarkets.

## The Real Food Pillars

Dr. Price also found a great variety in traditional diets, which were of course influenced by their geographic location. On the surface, the diets looked completely different. For example, the Inuit of Alaska had a completely different diet than the Masai tribe of Africa. Obviously, the Masai weren't hunting seals and whales, and the Inuit weren't about to raise cows on the frozen tundra. But the genius of Dr. Price was that he found, *underneath the surface,* that all native cultures had *similar principles* in preparing food despite living in vastly different climates. It's these unifying principles that weave and connect all dietary traditions throughout human history. They can also help us understand why we should be eating these foods and the roles they play in boosting our stomach acidity naturally and thus stopping heartburn.

I call these principles the "real food pillars," and we are going to discuss five of them in the five chapters that follow. In the process, we'll be taking a bit of a detour away from directly discussing heartburn and GERD. But it will all come full circle in Part III when we apply these five pillars in the 3-Step Plan. So be patient! Trust me—to start the 3-Step Plan right now would create a lot more questions than answers. With a thorough understanding of the five real food pillars, you will be much better prepared to start the 3-Step Plan and kiss heartburn and GERD goodbye once and for all.

# 6

# Say Goodbye to Low Fat

**R**eal Food Pillar #1: No culture on this planet *ever* ate a low-fat diet.

Dr. Price found every culture he studied valued healthy fats. Dairy was consumed raw and in whole form. No one ever drank skim milk. Animal fats such as lard, tallow, bacon fat, butter, poultry fat, and the fat from marine animals were used liberally. In fact, many of these fats were considered sacred for fertility and children's health. And those that tended towards plant-based diets in warm-weather climates regularly consumed healthy fats in the form of dairy, eggs, fish, coconuts, and palm oils.

**There is no greater nutritional myth than the idea that fat is bad for you.** Fat is to your body like oil is to your car. It keeps things lubricated and running smoothly and efficiently.

Here is a short list of what fat does in your body:

- provides the building blocks of cell membranes
- is required for the absorption of vitamins A, D, E, and K
- is necessary in the natural process of inflammation
- provides the building blocks for hormones, including testosterone and estrogen
- is necessary for mental health
- is a protective lining for organs

- is necessary for healthy skin, hair, and nails
- improves the digestion and absorption of food

Let's focus on that last one. Remember, it is the maldigestion of carbohydrates that gives off gases in the stomach that can build up pressure and contribute to food refluxing back into the esophagus. By reducing our carbohydrates significantly, especially in the first few weeks, and eating more healthy fats, we can stop this buildup of pressure.

## But Aren't Fats Bad for Us?

Of course, the conventional advice is to reduce fats to help heartburn. Fats, we're told, will make us fat, clog our arteries, and make us sick. But no one ever differentiates between good fats and bad fats.

The theory that fat is bad for us, causes weight gain, and clogs our arteries is known as the lipid hypothesis. Many people are surprised to learn that it is a theory, *not* a fact. In reality, countless studies have proven it wrong in recent years.[1,2,3] However, it continues to be pushed by corporate interests to sell processed foods. The food industry knows that no matter how much sugar, trans fats, chemicals, and preservatives they put in food, if they slap a low-fat label on it, sales increase.

*"The diet-heart hypothesis has been repeatedly shown to be wrong and yet, for complicated reasons of pride, profit, and prejudice, the hypothesis continues to be exploited by scientists, fundraising enterprises, food companies, and even governmental agencies. The public is being deceived by the greatest health scam of the century."*

- George Mann, former co-director of the Framingham Heart Study

The biggest difference between good and bad fats is *how they are processed*. Good fats occur naturally in nature. Bad fats do not occur naturally and are greatly changed via industrial processes.

| Good Fats | Bad Fats |
| --- | --- |
| Meat from wild or pastured animals | Meat from factory-farmed animals |
| Wild fish | Most farmed fish |
| Organic, pastured eggs | Eggs from factory-farmed chickens |
| Raw dairy | Pasteurized and homogenized dairy |
| Butter | Smart Balance or Earth Balance |
| Tropical oils – coconut oil, palm oil | Non-tropical oils exposed to heat |
| First cold pressed, extra virgin olive oil | Pure and/or refined olive oil |
| Whole nuts and seeds | Most nut and seed oils |

## Incredibly Bad Fats and the Quadruple Bypass

Right now, take a look at the products in your fridge and kitchen cabinets. Unless you're aware of this, I can almost guarantee you'll see corn, cottonseed, canola, and/or soybean oil in almost everything–salad dressings, mayonnaise, cookies, potato chips, canned goods, and even things like bread.

These are the *incredibly bad fats*. I call these four the "quadruple bypass" not just for their association with heart disease but also because any time you see these four oils in anything, bypass them! Crisco was introduced in 1911, and it was the first shortening made entirely of vegetable oil. Margarine soon followed. This is the time when the rates of heart disease started to dramatically escalate in industrialized countries.

The advent of TV and radio offered a wonderful marketing opportunity for the vegetable oil industry, and after World War II, almost every household in America was convinced that these oils were better for us than traditional fats. Traditional animal fats were replaced with products such as Mazola, Wesson, and PAM cooking sprays. Our food supply has been virtually saturated (no pun intended) by these heavily refined oils.

The food industry *loves* these oils because they are cheap and because they can be transformed into trans fats to make foods shelf-stable. However, these artificial fats are *devastating* to human health. The research connecting trans fats to chronic disease is about as solid as the research connecting cigarette smoking to lung cancer.

Trans fats are formed in a high-tech process called hydrogenation. This process turns liquid oils into solid fats. If you see the word "hydrogenated" on a food label, it is almost always one of the quadruple bypass oils. You'll often see two or more of them together as, for example, "partially hydrogenated corn and/or soybean oil."

These man-made fats are similar in structure to saturated fats but act very differently in the body. Unfortunately, trans fats and natural saturated fats are rarely differentiated in nutritional studies. Thus, saturated fats have been incorrectly blamed for every health problem under the sun.

This includes heartburn.

Eating the right types of fats is vital for digestive health and thus vital for stopping heartburn and resetting the acidity in your stomach. They are therefore an important part of the 3-Step Plan.

The topic of fats could easily be another book on its own. If you would like a more thorough overview of good fats and bad fats and the rise of incredibly bad fats in our food supply, please read the following excellent article by Dr. Mary Enig and Sally Fallon:

http://www.westonaprice.org/know-your-fats/the-oiling-of-america

# 7

# What Dietitians Don't Know About Whole Grains

**Real Food Pillar #2: Grains were properly prepared**

In the summer of 1999, I read a book called *A Diet for a New America* by John Robbins.

The premise of this book was that raising animals is not only unethical but also bad for the environment and bad for our health. Like most that grew up in the suburbs, I was completely disconnected from my food source. It was the first time I learned of the horrors of the industrial food system, and I wanted no part of it anymore. As a result, I became a vegetarian for the next seven years.

Of course, it wasn't until years later that I learned there is a great difference between the industrial system and the small-scale sustainable system of raising animals on pasture, as nature intended and as Dr. Price found in every traditional culture he studied. *A Diet for a New America* made no such distinction.

And so I did what most vegetarians do in America. I gave up meat thinking that was all I had to do to be healthy. I ate the health-conscious Standard American Diet. And one of the biggest tenets of the health-conscious Standard American Diet is this idea that for good health, you should eat lots of whole grains.

On the surface, it makes sense. When we look at the nutrients in whole grains, we see they contain protein, essential fats, minerals, antioxidants, and fiber. Sounds good, right?

And so I started eating A LOT of whole grains. Organic breakfast cereals and granola (with low-fat milk, of course), stir-fries, whole grain breads, and whole grain pasta dishes became my staples.

However, after a few years, I started developing digestive issues. In particular, I experienced chronic bloating. Food would just sit in my stomach for hours. Some days I'd wake up and the previous night's dinner would still be sitting there. I wasn't hungry again until dinner. I felt awful. Fatigue became my every day companion. I wasn't digesting and absorbing the nutrients in my food despite eating a mostly organic, whole foods diet.

Of course, nobody ever told me about the difference between properly and improperly prepared grains. Because nobody knew. My parents didn't know. My friends didn't know. Dietitians didn't know (and most still don't). My doctors had no idea. And John Robbins certainly didn't know either.

But Weston Price did.

Dr. Price found that those cultures that used grains were *very careful* in their preparation. Through hundreds if not thousands of years of trial and error and passed-down knowledge, these cultures knew that soaking, sprouting, and fermenting grains made them more digestible and healthier.

Laboratory analysis can identify a wide spectrum of beneficial nutrients in whole grains, but that doesn't mean our body utilizes them all, because there's something else in whole grains besides all those nutrients.

Anti-nutrients.

There's a reason you can store grains in containers in your kitchen for long periods without them rotting. Their outer shell prevents microbial breakdown and protects the nutrients inside. Under the right conditions, namely warmth, moisture, and time, a grain will sprout into a new plant. Herbivores such as cows and sheep have evolved a highly complex digestive system with multiple stomachs, long intestines, and a slow transit time that allow plants and grains to digest slowly so they can extract their nutrients.[1] In contrast, dogs and cats have only one stomach and cannot digest grains well. You'll never see a feral cat or wild dog in nature eating grains.

Humans too have a much simpler digestive system than herbivores. Like cats and dogs, humans also have only one stomach. But they also have a nice big brain, and they have figured out how to prepare plants in certain ways to maximize their digestibility. All traditional cultures had this knowledge.

Modern science confirms today that grains have something called phytic acid in their outer shell. This is what preserves grains for long periods. Phytic acid is an anti-nutrient that blocks mineral absorption in our intestines. However, soaking, sprouting, and fermenting grains neutralizes the phytic acid as well as several other anti-nutrients present in grains such as enzyme inhibitors, complex sugars, and complex proteins such as gluten. Furthermore, these methods *increase* the nutrient content of grains. They do this by mimicking the germination process that grains must go through to sprout into a new plant.[2]

Consuming large amounts of improperly treated grains can cause digestive problems. I am convinced this is what happened to me on a vegetarian diet.

A very trendy diet these days is the Paleo (short for Paleolithic) diet, which argues that humans were healthier before the advent of agriculture and civilization. Paleo diets remove all grains and remarkable transformations in health occur, especially when it comes to serious digestive conditions such as Crohn's disease, ulcerative colitis, chronic diarrhea, and IBS.

While I don't think we need to take all grains out of our diet forever, I do think limiting or even removing them for some time can be quite beneficial to allow our digestive system, including, of course, the acidity in our stomach, to reset. As you'll soon see, this is an important part of the 3-Step Plan.

8

# Make No Bones About It...

**R**eal Food Pillar #3: Almost every culture used bone broths.

Now, when I say bone broths, I mean REAL bone broths. Unfortunately, few Americans make real bone broths anymore. Instead, they use pre-prepared broths out of boxes and cans full of chemicals, preservatives, and artificial flavors. But even worse than that is the widespread use of bouillon cubes. One cube in some boiling water gets you an instant quasi-stock. But have you ever seen the ingredients label for most bouillon cubes? Here's is the ingredient label from one common product:

Salt, Sugar, Flavor (Hydrolyzed Soy Protein, Salt, Partially Hydrogenated Soy Oil), Hydrolyzed Soy Protein, Silicon Dioxide (Anticaking Agent), Fat Flavor (Partially Hydrogenated Corn Oil, Flavoring), Natural Flavor (Autolyzed Yeast Extract, Salt, Sugar, Whey Powder [from milk], Lactic Acid), Spice, Onion Powder, Dehydrated Cooked Beef, Caramel Color, Dried Beef Stock, Disodium Inosinate and Disodium Guanylate, Autolyzed Yeast, Flavoring. No MSG added (Contains Naturally Occurring Glutamates).

Let's just hit on a few of these nasty ingredients so I can hopefully scare you away from ever using these toxic little chemical cubes ever again.

At the top, you'll see partially hydrogenated soy oil and then on the next line, partially hydrogenated corn oil, two of the "quadruple bypass" ingredients.

Next you'll see "hydrolyzed soy protein," which is a soy byproduct that acts as a filler and flavor enhancer. It contains monosodium glutamate (MSG), which has been linked to headaches, muscle tightness, tingling sensations, and general weakness.[1]

Moving down, you'll see the ubiquitous "natural flavors." "Natural flavors" are made in labs. According to the FDA, since they are derived from naturally occurring substances, they can be legally termed "natural."[2] The purpose of natural flavors is flavoring, not nutrition.

Next you'll see the ingredient, "Spice." Hello?! What spice? No one really knows except the food manufacturer. By law, food companies can use "spice" or "spices" in the same way they use the term "natural flavors" to disguise a whole host of chemicals. Food companies do this to not only hide their chemical concoctions from the public but also to hide them from their competitors.

Make no mistake about it—these chemical formulas are big business. *Really big business*. And the food industry wants to keep their formulas a secret as much as possible. Deceptive labeling is the way they do this.

Moving down we see more chemicals. But the last one is my personal favorite, "No MSG added (contains *naturally occurring glutamates*)."

Here's a good explanation about the term "naturally occurring" from the website www.truthinlabeling.org:

"By FDA definition, processed free glutamic acid (MSG) is 'naturally occurring,' because the basic ingredients are found in nature. 'Naturally occurring' does not mean that a food additive is being used in its natural state. 'Naturally occurring' only means that the food additive began with something found in nature. By FDA definition, the ingredient 'monosodium glutamate' is natural. So is hydrochloric acid. So is arsenic. 'Natural' doesn't mean 'safe.'" [3]

And MSG can be hidden in many other sources, like, say, hydrolyzed soy protein.

Of course, it doesn't end with just bouillon cubes. Canned soups are just as bad and contain many of the same things to mimic the flavors found in real stocks and soups. If you have any Campbell's or Progresso soup in your cupboard at the moment, take a look at the ingredients. Or don't. Because you'll be horrified.

There's no denying canned soups and bouillon cubes are convenient. One of my favorite authors on real food even admits to using them every now and then when she's in a pinch. Luckily, cooking real stocks is one of the most convenient, simple, traditional foods you can prepare at home. Once you get into a habit of making them, the flavor, the versatility, and the health benefits will keep you from using the fake stuff except on the rarest of occasions.

## The Benefits of Real Bone Broth

Bone broths are basically just bones that are simmered in water for an extended period of time. This simmering leaches the nutrients out of the bones and presents them in a highly absorbable and thus digestible form.

*Dr. Price found every culture used the bones of their animals for making broths.* These broths formed the foundation of staples such as soups, gravies, stews, curries, tagines, bouillabaisses, cioppinos, and gumbos. They've been used for centuries for their restorative, immune-boosting power.

This is a lot more evident in other parts of the world. In my travels through Asia, steaming cauldrons of traditional soups were a common part of street fare, market stalls, and cafes. And grandma (or maybe great-grandma) may not be a scientist, but she's observed over and over how chicken soup helps one recover from the common cold. It is this repeated observation of a food's therapeutic benefit that traditional cultures understood.

They had thousands of years of trial and error; they did not need scientific studies to validate what to eat and why.

In particular, bone broths are loaded with minerals. Bone is made mostly of minerals, including calcium, magnesium, phosphorus, and other trace minerals, so the long application of heat and water will slowly draw them out. In fact, if you were to cook the bones long enough, they would crumble and even dissolve in the water. And minerals are not denatured like fats or proteins, so no matter how long you cook your broth, they will remain intact.

What does this have to do with heartburn and GERD, you might be asking?

## Mineral Deficiencies and Low Stomach Acid

I was watching TV the other day and, sure enough, a commercial came on for Nexium, aka "The Purple Pill." Nexium is a proton pump inhibitor, which, as mentioned previously, is the most powerful type of heartburn medication. One of the side effects mentioned on the commercial was increased risk of bone fracture and low magnesium.

Actually, this really isn't a side effect as much as it is a *direct effect* of taking PPIs. As we've seen, long-term use of heartburn medication lowers or, as in the case of PPIs, shuts down our stomach's acid production. But proper acid production is needed to extract the minerals from our food so that the minerals can be absorbed properly into the bloodstream.

Guess what happens when that acidity is compromised. That's right. Poor mineral absorption. I'm not sure why that commercial singled out just low magnesium as a side effect when studies show that iron, calcium, and zinc are also poorly absorbed in cases of hypochlorhydria. [4]

If that commercial had been more truthful, it would have also said that long-term use of antacids *increases the risk* of osteoporosis. [5,6] Osteoporosis is a condition in which the bones become weak and brittle due to a loss of minerals. According to the National Osteoporosis Foundation, there are approximately

44 million Americans with either osteoporosis or low bone mass, and this number is expected to skyrocket in the coming decades.[7]

Even the Food and Drug Administration required PPIs to carry new warning labels in 2010 regarding their association with mineral deficiencies and bone fractures.

"Epidemiology studies suggest a possible increased risk of bone fractures with the use of proton pump inhibitors for one year or longer, or at high doses. Because these products are used by a great number of people, it's important for the public to be aware of this possible increased risk..."[8] (Joyce Korvick, M.D., deputy director for safety in FDA's Division of Gastroenterology Products)

Considering that one in five Americans is taking some form of acid-suppressing drug, it stands to reason that the high rates of heartburn and GERD may be contributing to this disturbing trend. Certainly, our modern agricultural methods, which deplete the soil of minerals, and the widespread consumption of processed foods play significant roles as well.

## The Problem with TUMS and Mineral Supplementation

Many who take acid-suppressing medications are aware of the connection to mineral deficiencies and seek out mineral supplementation. Because of the growing trends in osteoporosis, even the FDA, which is often opposed to taking supplements, recommends calcium supplementation.

One of the more bizarre results of all this is the common medical advice to take TUMS for calcium. The active ingredient in TUMS is calcium carbonate, which temporarily alkalinizes stomach acid. While this works to temporarily stop heartburn, over the long term, it compromises the body's ability to absorb minerals, including the very mineral it's prescribed for. *The irony in this is both tragic and comical at the same time!*

Other mineral supplements may not be that much better. It is highly controversial whether or not our bodies even utilize the minerals in supplement form. Elemental, chelated, ionic, and colloidal forms of minerals are all available in supplement form. Of course, all the supplement manufacturers claim their products are the most absorbable, but wouldn't you if your income was dependent upon it?

And yet we know minerals are highly available to us in whole food form where they are combined with other molecules present in foods that allow them to be digested properly. Minerals don't exist in a vacuum. They coexist and work synergistically with other nutrients. We are so conditioned to think that a drug or overpriced supplement is a quick fix to solve our health problems that few even consider improving their diet. We all know that few doctors counsel their patients in nutrition. Even many integrative and holistic healthcare practitioners prescribe supplements first before even discussing dietary changes.

Well, not here. In this book, you are learning about the power of REAL food. Supplements are always secondary to dietary changes in my book (pun intended). And as you'll see, supplements are often completely unnecessary.

Bone broths are about as real as it gets. They are one of the easiest ways to insure a healthy supply of easily absorbable minerals, especially if you've been on acid-blocking medications for an extended period of time. If this is the case, there can be some initial digestive difficulties when introducing more traditional foods. Bone broths will help tremendously in the early stages of that transition. But bone broths do a lot more than just supply the body with minerals. After all, bone broths are a whole food. In Chapter 12, you'll learn about a few other nutrients in bone broths that will specifically aid your recovery from heartburn and GERD.

For now, let's move on to the fourth real food pillar.

# 9

# To Drink Milk or Not to Drink Milk?

**R**eal Food Pillar #4: Real milk is *raw* milk

To drink milk, or not to drink milk. Ask a hundred people and you'll get a hundred different answers. Find a hundred studies on the health effects of drinking milk and you'll get a hundred different results, both good and bad.

Naysayers say humans are the only animal that drinks the milk from another animal, that cow's milk is food for baby cows, that milk is high in saturated fat and cholesterol, that milk is hard to digest, contains antibiotics and growth hormones, and can contribute to asthma and allergic reactions. And all of this is true! Just ask anyone who's taken dairy out of their diet and experienced better health.

Enthusiasts say milk is a good source of calcium and other minerals, beneficial bacteria, protein, enzymes, healthy fats, and vitamin A and D, and can contribute to strong bones and help *prevent* asthma and allergies. Also true. Just ask those who have included *more* dairy in their diet and experienced better health as a result.

So who's right?

Again, it comes down to *the source* of the milk. Not all milk is created equal.

The naysayers never—**and I mean NEVER**—distinguish between the milk you find in supermarkets and real milk. Real milk is *raw* milk that comes from pastured cows that eat their natural diet of grass. This is the milk the enthusiasts are talking about. Please keep in mind that the words "raw" and "milk" have only been used together in recent times to differentiate raw milk from modern milk. Traditionally, raw milk was just called "milk" in the same way that "organic food" was just called "food."

Today, the word "raw" scares people because of the possibility of exposure to pathogenic bacteria, but the risk of contracting a food-borne illness from raw milk is minute compared to other foods. According to the CDC, from 1996 to 2003, there were 46 outbreaks due to raw milk and ZERO deaths. Let me repeat that. ZERO deaths.[1]

Contrast that to the average of 3,000 deaths, 128,000 hospitalizations, and 48 million gastrointestinal illnesses that occur every year due to food-borne illnesses.[2] The overwhelming majority of these come from large-scale industrial models of food production. In recent years, major food recalls have become almost commonplace. Lettuce, spinach, alfalfa, beef, and even cantaloupes have sickened thousands.[3]

Make no mistake about it. Raw milk is a major threat to the conventional dairy industry, which has convinced our government that raw milk is unsafe and has worked behind the scenes to pass laws to make raw milk illegal or difficult to access in most states. Scare tactics in the media have now evolved to actual physical scare tactics as the federal and state governments have started armed raids on many small raw dairy farms across the country.

In many ways, these attacks on raw milk represent the growing divide between our "grow food at whatever cost necessary to public and environmental health" food system and Americans' growing awareness and demand for food grown locally and sustainably.

A rising tide of documentaries, books, and blogs are lifting the veil on the horrors of industrialized food to the American public.

There is probably no better example of that than the conditions and treatments of modern milk.

Let's understand three reasons why.

### Reason #1: CAFOs

Concentrated Animal Feeding Operations (CAFOs) is the politically correct term for factory farms that began to uproot the traditional family farm in the 1930s.

CAFOs have become the predominant method of raising animals in the US and many other industrialized countries since World War II. The CAFO model confines animals into small spaces to maximize their potential for growth and thus profits.

Cows in CAFOs are fed grains and soybeans, which fatten them more quickly than grass. They're also given growth hormones to encourage further milk production. But this is not their natural diet, and it changes milk's nutrient profile. It is also not uncommon for CAFO cows to be fed other industry byproducts such as bakery waste, cottonseed meal, chicken manure, and even the remains of dead slaughterhouse animals. Not surprisingly, this unnatural diet makes them sick, for which they're then given antibiotics.[4] Because they're not out on pasture, their manure accumulates quickly, causing incredibly unsanitary conditions that pose risks to the environment, the cows themselves, and, of course, to us.

### Reason #2: Pasteurization and homogenization

These filthy conditions have led to the industry-wide adoption of pasteurization. Pasteurization heats milk to a high temperature, killing any potential pathogens. The dairy industry and the FDA say that pasteurization is a safety issue, that it's necessary to protect the public. And to a degree, I agree with this. I would *never* drink raw milk from CAFOs. Nor should you. However, milk was never intended to come from cows raised in filthy CAFOs.

The problem with pasteurization is that it kills a lot more than just pathogens. It also denatures the proteins and destroys the nutrients in milk, including the vitamins, enzymes, and the healthy bacteria. It leaves behind a highly nutrient-deficient product. This is the milk the overwhelming majority of Americans have been drinking since pasteurization became standard practice in the decades following World War II.

To add insult to injury, the dairy industry also employs the practice of homogenization. This technique blasts apart the fat molecules in milk under high pressure and re-suspends them in the milk. Most people today, having grown up on supermarket milk, have no idea that under normal conditions the fat in milk will rise to the surface. This is the cream used for things like butter and sour cream.

But unlike pasteurization, homogenization is not required by law. The dairy industry does it simply to create a more uniform looking product, which of course is good for business.

## Osteoporosis and Digestibility

This newfangled modern dairy is causing major problems in our ability to digest it. I've encountered countless people who claim major improvements in health when they take out dairy for a while. As just a few examples, chronic constipation dissipates, chronic sinus issues clear, acne fades, and even heartburn symptoms improve. *Of course, what they're taking out is modern dairy, not traditional raw milk.*

But the one health issue that's interesting to look at in particular is osteoporosis because of the widespread belief that the calcium in milk is good for your bones. Both raw and pasteurized milk have similar levels of minerals, but high heat alters the fat-soluble vitamins that are necessary in order to absorb and utilize the minerals in the water portion of milk. Furthermore, it also alters the enzymes that help us absorb the minerals.

Mark McAfee, champion of raw milk and owner of Organic Pastures Dairy, a raw milk dairy in California, writes:

"It has long been known by doctors that low-fat pasteurized milk is a real problem when considering bone density and osteoporosis. The test for pasteurization is called the negative alpha phosphatase test. When milk has been heated to 165 degrees and pasteurization is complete, the enzyme phosphatase is 100 percent destroyed. Guess what? This is the enzyme that is critical for the absorption of minerals including calcium! Phosphatase is the third most abundant enzyme in raw milk and those who drink raw milk enjoy increased bone density. Several studies have documented greater bone density and longer bones in animals and humans consuming raw milk compared to pasteurized." [5]

The United States has one of the highest rates of milk consumption in the world and yet one of the highest rates of osteoporosis. Again, few doctors, ZERO major health organizations, and certainly not anyone behind the dairy industry-funded "Got Milk?" campaign is telling you the difference between conventional and raw milk. Well-paid and perhaps well-intentioned celebrities with milk mustaches probably don't know the difference either.

Consider that none of the raw-milk-drinking cultures Dr. Price studied experienced the wide range of problems that many do today on modern milk. And though Dr. Price could not measure bone density, he always noted excellent teeth (which is bone) and physical structure in all of the cultures he studied.

Even more interestingly, raw milk used to have a role in *helping* various digestive disturbances, *including heartburn*. More about that in Chapter 12.

### Reason #3: Low-fat milk

If you're old enough, you may remember your mother or grandmother bemoaning the lack of flavor in the store-bought milk that was starting to supplant the raw milk from the local family farms. If you have access to raw milk, compare the difference in taste. It's shockingly obvious, especially for a reason besides pasteurization.

**Real milk is not low-fat milk!** Perhaps that's why nature designed fats to taste good? Everyone knows that low-fat products don't taste as good. It's both tragic and comedic to think that that we have become so conditioned to be afraid of fat that we will actually consume low-fat products full of chemicals and sugar before real, whole foods with healthy fats. Think margarine over butter; sugary low-fat yogurt over whole milk yogurt; toxic vegetable oils over traditional fats like coconut oil, lard, and tallow; and of course, skim milk over whole milk.

The fats in milk provide more than just flavor. *They also provide essential nutrients.* In particular, it's where the vitamin A and D are located. Vitamin A and D are fat-soluble vitamins, meaning they need fat to be absorbed in the body. Furthermore, most people think milk is a good source of minerals, especially calcium. And it is. But did you know that vitamin A and D help you absorb the minerals in milk? This is why Dr. Price never found any culture ever drinking skim or low-fat milk.

## Raw Milk Benefits

Raw milk is the milk that cultures have used ever since humans started domesticating animals thousands of years ago. Dr. Weston Price found milk from cows, sheep, and goats to be an integral part of the diets of many of the cultures he encountered. Other cultures used the milk from camels, water buffaloes, reindeer, and yaks. Keeping and caring for these animals proved an excellent survival strategy in more rugged landscapes not suitable to tillable soil.

Certainly, this widespread and varied use of milk throughout human history indicates a nutritional benefit! Humans have indeed adapted the ability to digest milk from other animals. Lactase, the enzyme that splits milk's double sugar, lactose, is present in all human babies but fades with weaning. Those that are lactose intolerant lack lactase and thus cannot digest milk. However, scientists estimate that somewhere around 10,000 years ago, some humans developed a genetic mutation that kept lactase hanging around after infancy. This mutation spread across Europe, Asia, and other areas of the world and allowed humans to drink milk throughout life.[6]

This ability to digest milk conferred enormous benefits to humans. From a nutritional standpoint, raw, whole milk is a complete food. Here is a short list of some of the nutrients in raw milk:

- Fat-soluble vitamins, A, D, E, and K
- Water-soluble vitamins, C, B6, and B12
- Minerals including calcium, magnesium, potassium, copper, selenium, and iron
- Conjugated linoleic acid (CLA), a fatty acid that's been shown to help with weight loss and has anti-cancer properties
- All eight essential amino acids
- Beneficial bacteria—vital for good intestinal health and protects against pathogens
- Enzymes to promote digestibility

As we've seen, poor quality feed, pasteurization, and removing the milk fat dramatically alter those nutrients and impact their digestibility.

To make a long story short, modern milk that is sold in supermarkets is a vastly different product than raw milk that comes from grass-fed cows. What I've included here is just the tip of the iceberg. If you'd like to learn more, including a list of raw milk dairies by state, please visit www.realmilk.com.

# 10

# Why You Should Eat More Bugs (not What You Think)

**R**eal Food Pillar #5: Every culture ate fermented foods

OK, back to my free initial consult with potential clients. Remember the quiet head nods I described after saying that I work with real food?

It's funny how quickly those agreeable head nods turn to quizzical looks when I start to delve deeper into what I mean by real food. Fats, bone broths, and properly prepared grains are not exactly what their doctor is telling them to eat. And when I mention that real food also includes fermented foods, I'd say about half the people say, "Ummm...what are fermented foods?"

Most people eat more of them than they realize. The four most common ones in America are probably cheese, yogurt, pickles, and sauerkraut.

I don't know about you, but growing up, the only fermented vegetables I ever ate were Vlasic pickles and sauerkraut. God how I *loooooved* those Vlasic pickles. If my parents had let me, I could've eaten the entire jar in one sitting. The sauerkraut? Not so much. I don't think I ever once tasted fresh sauerkraut in my childhood. My parents, probably like most suburban parents in the 70s and 80s, bought it in cans solely for its use as a topping on hot dogs.

As for fermented dairy, while I ate my fair share of overly sweetened yogurts with chemicals and high-fructose corn syrup, my personal favorite was American cheese. To this day, it is still my favorite cheese. I can't tell you how many omelets and grilled cheese sandwiches I ate overloaded with it. Probably took a few years off my life. But when I learned that American cheese isn't really cheese but a highly processed product full of emulsifiers, colorings, and even corn syrup, I immediately stopped eating it. In fact, I stopped eating a lot of cheese that I found in the supermarket.

Just like the other real food pillars, not all fermented foods are created equal. They need to be *properly fermented* to be truly fermented. Neither the Vlasic pickles nor the canned sauerkraut nor the Dannon yogurt and certainly not the American cheese were properly fermented. Unfortunately, this goes for just about every so-called fermented food in your supermarket.

### Back to the Bacteria

Remember, the digestive system, especially the large intestine, is populated by trillions of bacteria. Proper fermentation is about encouraging those healthy bacteria to proliferate in food. On purpose.

That may sound creepy in our antibacterial obsessed world, but it is these bacteria that are vital to the health of our digestive system, including the resolution of heartburn.

These bacteria are not only present inside us; they're also present outside. They live on the surface of all living things (including us), and they are especially abundant on the roots and leaves of plants. Proper fermentation manipulates conditions to allow these bacteria to break down the starches and sugars in fruits and vegetables as well as dairy and convert them into lactic acid. Thus, fermentation is also referred to as lacto-fermentation. This lactic acid inhibits pathogenic bacteria and preserves food and prevents spoilage. It's also what gives fermented foods their notoriously sour flavor. It's how we get pickles from cucumbers, sauerkraut from cabbage, and the myriad of fermented milk products such as cheese, yogurt, and kefir.

Along the way, as the bacteria feed on the sugars, they also multiply.

Properly fermented foods are ALIVE, teeming with billions upon billions of those bacteria that populate our digestive tract. So when we eat fermented foods, they act as a raft for bacteria to move into our gut and take up residence where they play some remarkable roles in keeping us healthy.

Here are just a few ways these bacteria keep us healthy:

- Enhance digestibility
- Increase vitamin content, in particular B vitamins and vitamins C and K
- Improve mineral absorption, including calcium
- Produce helpful digestive enzymes
- Produce anticarcinogenic substances
- Produce butyric acid, which promotes healthy colon function
- Promote immune system health
- Lower cholesterol
- Protect against bone loss

These healthy bacteria go by another name you may have heard: probiotics.

Probiotic translates to "pro-life." Many people today take probiotics in supplement form. These supplements are formulated in laboratories and contain bacteria that occur naturally in our digestive system, particularly our large intestine. The word "antibiotics" translates to "anti-life" and they are prescribed by doctors to kill harmful bacteria within us. While this may be necessary at times, antibiotics don't discriminate and also kill the beneficial bacteria. This is why probiotic supplements are often used after a round of antibiotics to repopulate the gut with good, health-promoting bacteria. As beneficial as these supplements can be, cultured foods are nature's true probiotics. Cheaper too.

Dr. Price found every culture he encountered consuming fermented foods. And not just for their health benefits. Remember, the lactic acid in these foods acts as a preservative so these foods were more common before the advent of refrigeration. If you're old enough, you may still remember your parents or grandparents preparing large crocks of sauerkraut in the fall and storing them in a root cellar for the winter.

Unfortunately, proper fermentation went out the window with the rise of processed foods.

## Vinegar and Pasteurization

In the decades after World War II, the use of vinegar and pasteurization became standard industry practice. Just like with milk, the politically correct reason is "safety," but the real reason is increased shelf life and a more uniform product.

Adding vinegar and pasteurizing sterilizes and preserves fermented foods for long periods of time. Vinegar has the added bonus of mimicking the sour flavor of fermented foods and creating a more consistent product taste-wise. Now instead of needing proper storage in cool conditions, they could be transported more easily and then stored on shelves for years upon years. But pasteurization and the use of vinegar kill the beneficial bacteria, which is the very point of consuming fermented foods!

Grandma and grandpa's root cellar was now on its way to becoming entertainment-filled furnished basements in the rapidly growing suburbs of America.

## How to Find Traditionally Fermented Foods

The good news in all of this is that unlike milk, it's not illegal to produce and sell properly fermented foods. I am incredibly lucky to live in an area where we have a wonderful local company that produces a line of traditionally fermented vegetables. You might have one in your area, too. If not, there are usually many good companies in your local health food stores. Always read the labels and make sure there is no vinegar or pasteurization used.

The one exception would be dairy. Though you can find raw cheeses in stores, most store-bought fermented dairy is pasteurized. However, if you see "contains live cultures" on the label, that means the company added good bacteria after pasteurization. You'll see this frequently on better quality yogurts. You can also check out the heartburn resources page on my website for a list of companies that make good quality fermented foods: http://fearlesseating.net/heartburn-book-resources

# Part III

## The 3-Step Plan

# The Steps:

**Step 1:** Go grain-free for the first two weeks.

**Step 2:** Soothe and repair the digestive tract with the five real food pillars for the entire four weeks.

**Step 3:** Soothe and repair the digestive tract with supplementation in the second two weeks but *only if necessary*.

# 11

# Against the Grain

**S**tep #1 - Go grain-free for the first two weeks.

In alternative circles, it's well established that going on a low-carbohydrate diet can dramatically restore upper GI function.[1] It's also well established that a low carbohydrate diet is better for losing weight and for improving metabolic risk factors such as total cholesterol, HDL cholesterol (good), LDL cholesterol (bad), triglycerides, fasting blood sugar, and blood pressure.[2,3,4,5]

A low-carbohydrate diet basically means reducing or even completely eliminating starches and sugars from refined grains and refined sugar. Low-carb diets emphasize fat- and protein-based meals and snacks with carbohydrates from mostly fruits and vegetables. Moderate amounts of whole grains and legumes are often included as well.

For our purposes, I want you to go a little further than just going low carb. I want you to remove *all grains*, including whole grains, for two weeks. This almost ensures you'll be doing a low-carb diet, as grains are the primary culprit in the standard American high-carb diet. But going grain-free also means you'll be doing three other things at the same time that are specific to stopping acid reflux.

**1. You'll be doing a gluten-free trial.**

A doctor I met a while ago said, "If you do nothing for your patients other than get them off wheat, 50% will come back and thank you." Now that's a dramatic statement! Let's understand why.

Take a look around your grocery store and you'll notice a new section that's not only becoming more common, but also growing rapidly. It's called the gluten-free section. Gluten is a protein in wheat, rye, and barley. It's a very complex protein and difficult for the body to break down and digest. And it is collectively wreaking havoc in our bodies right now.

Nobody knows exactly why gluten is causing such widespread problems, but a growing consensus is pointing the finger at the dramatic changes wheat has undergone in recent decades. Cardiologist Dr. William Davis in his book *Wheat Belly* explains:

"So why has this seemingly benign plant that sustained generations of humans suddenly turned on us? For one thing, it is not the same grain our forebears ground into their daily bread. Wheat naturally evolved to only a modest degree over the centuries, but it has changed dramatically in the past fifty years under the influence of agricultural scientists. Wheat strains have been hybridized, crossbred, and introgressed to make the wheat plant resistant to environmental conditions, such as drought, or pathogens, such as fungi...

"The result: A loaf of bread, biscuit, or pancake of today is different than its counterpart of a thousand years ago, different even from what our grandmothers made. They might look the same, even taste much the same, but there are biochemical differences. Small changes in wheat protein structure can spell the difference between a devastating immune response to wheat protein versus no immune response at all...

"Wheat gluten proteins, in particular, undergo considerable structural change with hybridization. In one hybridization experiment, fourteen new gluten proteins were identified in the offspring that were not present in either parent wheat plant. Moreover, when compared to century-old strains of wheat, modern strains of *Triticum aestivum* (wheat) express a higher quantity of genes for gluten proteins that are associated with celiac disease."[6]

The overwhelming majority of the wheat grown in the world today, including organic, are these newer hybridized strains that have a higher gluten content than traditional strains.

And of course the food industry loves these new strains as they can morph wheat into any number of cheap, convenience foods—cereals, bread, cookies, snack products, pasta, muffins, pastries, bagels, etc. It has become a central part of most Americans' diet for this reason. And this is exacerbated by the often well-intentioned but misguided health advice to eat lots of whole grains, which as we've seen, are rarely properly prepared for optimal digestion.

More than 2 million Americans or 1 in 133 people have celiac disease, a diagnosed allergy to gluten.[7] But you don't have to have celiac disease to have a problem digesting gluten. The more common scenario, which is unknowingly affecting millions of people, is to have a gluten intolerance or sensitivity. This presents as a less obvious reaction to gluten and can be difficult to determine. Chronic, nagging health issues such as migraines, joint pain, fatigue, weight gain, mental fogginess, IBS, and, yes, heartburn are common symptoms. The best way to determine if you have a gluten sensitivity is to remove it for at least one month.

*Sometimes, that's all it takes to stop heartburn, and often it will resolve very quickly.*

"I'd had heartburn for 20 plus years. Popped TUMS and antacids like they were candy. Craig told me to start by removing gluten from my diet. Almost overnight, my heartburn disappeared. I couldn't believe it. I haven't touched an antacid since and better yet, my heartburn hasn't returned. Craig also taught me how to eat in a way that not only will support my digestive health but my overall health for years to come." - Eric L.

## 2. You'll stop eating a lot of refined carbohydrates and sugar.

And as we've learned, sugar and refined carbs can contribute to bacterial overgrowth and the production of excess gas in the intestines. Their overconsumption often leads to weight gain and many other common health problems.

Granted, you can still eat a lot of sugar on a grain-free diet, but it's amazing just how much sugar is doused on grain-based products. Cereals, muffins, cookies, cakes, and a seemingly infinite number of grain-based snack products, including "healthy" ones like granola bars, are often loaded with refined sugars. And yes, that includes gluten-free products too. This is often one of the common pitfalls of a gluten-free diet.

Of course, there are other ways to sneak sugar into our diets beyond just sugary grain products. So please be aware that refined sugar needs to be strictly limited if not completely eliminated during this two-week trial period. If you are a sugar addict, a growing and very real concern today, following Step 2 will greatly reduce your sugar cravings. This should also help tremendously if you need to lose weight.

> *"I'd been on an acid-blocker for many years and was about twenty pounds overweight. Craig introduced me to a low-carb approach, which was almost the exact opposite of what my doctor had been recommending. I took sugar out of my diet, reduced grains, and started eating more healthy fats and protein. Not only did my heartburn fade away but so did those excess pounds. Best of all, it was so easy. I never once experienced hunger or cravings."*
> - Joe K.

## 3. You'll stop eating improperly prepared grains.

As previously discussed, this will remove a great burden from your digestive system for a few weeks. At the same time, in Step 2, you'll be using real food to restore proper function in the three phases of your digestive system—the upper, middle, and lower GI tracts.

> *"In 2007 I was diagnosed with GERD. My doctor immediately put me on Prevacid. After a few years, it stopped working and I was switched to Nexium. In 2011, I met with Craig and I wasn't prepared for the scope of good advice that he gave me. I had no idea how much sugar I was eating—in juice, yogurt, and in cereal. Slowly, I began to look at the labels on products and make better choices. He also suggested I cut grains out of my diet for a while as well. I couldn't believe how good I felt after just a few weeks. After four years on acid blockers I quit taking them and have not felt the need for them since."*
> - Janice B.

## How to Go Grain-Free

If a grain-free diet sounds intimidating, don't freak out! It's not as hard as you think. Nor is it as restrictive as you think. We are not limiting caloric consumption here or doing any sort of "diet" in the conventional sense. I want you to eat well to nourish your body and your digestive system.

Essentially, for these first two weeks you'll be eating mostly fats and protein from meats, eggs, and dairy (if tolerated) with lots of homemade soups, vegetables, and fermented vegetables. Fruits, nuts, and legumes are allowed as well. Part IV will help you get started with recipes and lots of grain-free meal ideas for breakfast, lunch, dinner, and snacks.

If you're still freaking out at the prospect of going grain-free, know that millions of people all over the world are experiencing great benefits from going gluten- and grain-free. The first few days and weeks can certainly be challenging as you navigate through social situations, work situations, and new recipes and habits. But with a little planning, patience, and practice, it does become easier over time.

The information presented here is just the basics to get you going. If you feel you need more help with eliminating grains, there are many online support groups, forums, and blogs that can help you in the process. I've included some resources on my heartburn resources page: http://fearlesseating.net/heartburn-book-resources

## What Should I Do After Two Weeks?

The most important thing is to check in with how you're feeling. If things are going great and your symptoms of acid reflux are gone, then you can consider reintroducing grains. If things are improving but symptoms still persist, you should consider keeping grains out for a longer period of time. Also, it's important to consider the degree of your symptoms. If you have a more chronic, long-term case of heartburn with other associated digestive problems, you should consider keeping grains out for a longer period of time. Let your intuition guide you. And by all means, if your symptoms are gone but you're feeling so good that you want to continue going grain-free, that's perfectly fine too! Reintroduce grains when you feel ready.

When you do decide to bring grains back, here's what I recommend:

**1. Start with non-gluten grains.**

| Grains That Contain Gluten: | Gluten-Free Grains: |
|---|---|
| Wheat | Corn |
| Rye | Rice |
| Barley | Quinoa |
| Spelt | Millet |
| Kamut | Teff |
| Bulgur | Amaranth |
| Couscous | Sorghum |
| Triticale | Buckwheat |
| *Oats | *Oats |

**\*Note: Oats don't inherently contain gluten but are often cross-contaminated with gluten due to processing. Only purchase oats that are labeled "gluten-free."**

The easiest non-gluten grains to reintroduce are rice and oats as they are a common part of most Americans' diet and are readily available in all health food stores. Other non-gluten-containing grains include quinoa, amaranth, teff, millet, and buckwheat (despite the name). *Reintroduce them in moderation.* Start with a little oatmeal for breakfast or some rice with dinner. See how you feel. If your heartburn immediately returns, this is a sign you'll need to keep them out for a longer period of time. Most people are able to handle this step, though.

To help improve their digestibility, be sure to soak the grains overnight. To soak grains, cover them with warm water and add an acidic medium, like a squeeze of lemon or a teaspoon or two of yogurt or whey. This will help accelerate the breakdown of phytic acid and thus improve the digestibility. This is less necessary for white rice as the bran has already been removed. Cover and leave overnight. There's no need to drain the water though some say it improves the flavor. Draining or not, you might have to add more water during cooking.

## A Word About Oatmeal

I can't believe what passes as oatmeal in this country. People are either trudging their way through some tasteless, goopy, instant crap because it's "low in fat and cholesterol," or they're eating some packaged version with "natural flavors" and tons of sugar and chemicals.

There's no reason for either. Purchase oatmeal in whole form as either rolled oats or steel cut. Do not buy instant oatmeal, which is more processed. You can make oatmeal instant by soaking it overnight. This is also more nutritious. Add one part oats to two parts water and add a teaspoon of yogurt or whey or a squeeze of lemon. Simply heat in the morning and add more water if necessary. It will cook up very quickly though steel-cut oats will take a little longer than rolled oats.

Oatmeal should taste delicious! Healthy fats will make it more palatable and digestible. Add a heaping tablespoon of butter, a dollop of cream, coconut oil, or coconut flakes and top with whole milk yogurt. Add in some almonds or walnuts. If you need some sweetness, add in fruit and/or a dollop of raw honey or maple syrup. Sea salt to taste. I often add ALL of the above.

## 2. Reintroduce gluten-containing grains.

If things are going well with non-gluten-containing grains, you can consider reintroducing gluten. I would wait an additional two weeks though so that you really give yourself a full month off of gluten. A full 30-day gluten-free challenge is considered the gold standard for diagnosing gluten sensitivities as laboratory testing is not completely reliable.

After 30 days, eat anything with wheat in it—bread, muffins, a bagel—a few times a day for a few days, then stop and see how you feel for up to three days afterwards. If your heartburn returns, that's a solid indication that you're gluten intolerant.

Now you know gluten is a major factor. Best to keep it out for a much longer period of time, if not forever. But pay close attention to other issues as well—joint pain, headaches, intestinal pain, body rashes, etc. If any of those vanished in the first month and then return after eating wheat, that's another good sign you're gluten intolerant. Gluten sensitivities don't always present as digestive problems. In either of the above cases, you should return to a gluten-free diet.

**What If I'm OK with Gluten and Grains?**

Hopefully you can handle some grains after a few weeks and perhaps even some gluten after a month. If so, don't start rejoicing yet! This is not a license to return to the heavily grain-based Standard American Diet. *Keep grains in moderation from here on out.* Consume them with healthy fats and protein. Stay away from heavily processed, sugary wheat products.

If you do consume wheat, seek out more traditional strains of wheat such as einkorn, faro, and spelt. These have not been hybridized to the degree that modern gluten-containing grains have been and many people report they can digest them without problems—in moderation, of course. Properly prepared sourdough breads and sprouted grains breads, which are common in most health food stores, are also good choices.

See my heartburn resources page for some companies and products that use ancient grains and/or properly prepared modern grains.

# 12

# Where the Rubber Hits the Road

**S**tep #2 - Soothe and repair the digestive tract with the five real food pillars for the entire four weeks.

Step 1 will hopefully ease the burden of heartburn. It may even bring it to a screeching halt. And that's fantastic. But Step 2 is where the rubber really hits the road, because beyond just removing triggers, Step 2 will start to reverse the years of acid reflux as well as the associated problems of low stomach acid.

This chapter should make A LOT more sense now that you have a good understanding of real food. And it should make EVEN MORE SENSE now that you have a better understanding of how the digestive system works and why heartburn occurs. Now we're going to apply the real food pillars to each of the three sections of the digestive tract, going once again from north to south. In doing so, you'll soothe and repair your digestive system so that you not only stop heartburn and GERD but you lay the foundation for it to NEVER return.

Now if you only have a mild case of heartburn, then I'm very confident that going grain-free in combination with the first step below will be all it takes to stop it. However, I'm going to take an educated guess and say that you probably have more than a mild case. Heartburn is so common these days that most folks brush it off as a normal part of life. That is, until it becomes chronic and starts to impact their quality of life. Unfortunately, most wait until this stage to seek help. If that describes you, the rest of this program will be very helpful to reverse years of damage to not only the esophagus but more than likely to other parts of the digestive system.

## 1. The upper GI – Part I

**Support the stomach (boost the blender speed) with healthy fats and protein while going grain-free.**

In combination with going grain-free for two weeks, increasing your intake of fat and protein will dramatically help restore your stomach's acidity. This is somewhat implied in Step 1, but it's a good reinforcement of why fats and protein will be so beneficial both now and over the long run.

Remember, protein is needed to *drive digestion*. Pepsin, the enzyme in our stomach that digests our proteins, is activated by hydrochloric acid. It works synergistically with HCl. Therefore, *protein needs strong acid production to work properly.*

Good quality fats have anti-inflammatory properties and will help soothe the lining of your stomach and intestines. They will also reduce cravings for sugar and refined carbs as you will feel fuller for longer periods between meals.

Perhaps there's a reason that fats and protein occur together in nature so often. And this is why *good quality* animal foods are such great sources of nutrition. They contain a full complement of amino acids and are an excellent source of healthy fats.

So what that means is *no more low-fat foods. Ever.* Better yet, that also means no more fake fat foods. No more margarine, Smart Balance, I Can't Believe It's Not Butter, Olivio, or any other product that makes you think it's better than good old-fashioned butter. Please throw them out immediately!

*Just. Eat. Butter.*

That's right, I want you to eat full fat foods, and I want you to eat healthy protein. Are your taste buds already dancing with anticipation and excitement? Before we got terribly confused about nutrition in the twentieth century, our taste buds were nature's way of telling us what to eat and why. Think about it, do you really like skim milk more than whole milk? Do you really like margarine more than butter? Do you really like a dry, lean cut of meat more than a juicy, marbled one?

Of course not.

**Examples of Healthy Protein**

- Wild caught and/or sustainably raised seafood
- Grass-fed beef
- Grass-fed lamb
- Wild game
- Pastured poultry
- Pastured eggs
- Pastured pork
- Raw dairy
- Cultured dairy – yogurt, kefir, cheese, sour cream, crème fraiche
- Raw nuts and seeds, soaked
- Legumes, properly prepared

**Note: Part IV will help you put this all together with recipe and meal ideas. In the meantime, let's cover some common obstacles and concerns when applying these real food pillars.**

**Troubleshooting**

**But Protein and Fat Make Me Feel Bloated!**

After years, if not decades, of eating the Standard American Diet, it is not uncommon for some to initially experience digestive discomfort when transitioning to a low-carb diet. Gas, bloating, heaviness, nausea, and, yes, heartburn may manifest.

Low fat, no fat, or poor quality fat will greatly impact your body's ability to digest it. Not eating fat is like never adding oil to the engine of your car. Eventually things are going to get gunked up. Time and time again, I see people on restricted fat diets lose their gallbladder. The gallbladder's job is to store and release bile to digest fats, but it does so *only in the presence of fat*. In fact, there's a common expression when it comes to our gallbladder: **Use it or lose it!** You absolutely need healthy fats to keep your gallbladder working properly.

Same for protein. You need protein to be able to digest protein. Years of low-protein or poor quality protein in conjunction with a high-carb diet can greatly compromise your stomach's acidity. And when you compromise the acidity, you also compromise pepsin, the enzyme necessary to begin digesting proteins.

Modern-day vegetarians are a perfect example. I see SO MANY vegetarians in my practice that have major digestive issues. Again, this is not because vegetarianism is inherently unhealthy but rather, just like myself, so many go about it so horribly wrong. Vegetarians that return to eating meat often complain of feeling sick to their stomach initially.

There are two things you can do if eating more fat and protein makes you feel worse.

The first is to be patient and push through. Most find their body adjusts within a few days, and they start to feel better. If eating fat makes you feel bloated, try using some coconut oil. You can use it as a cooking oil, put it on your vegetables, or put it in a smoothie. Coconut oil contains lots of medium chain triglycerides, a type of saturated fat that is very easy on the body's digestion. You could even use it as supplement and take a teaspoon or two per day away from food. And if you struggle with overeating, try taking a little coconut oil about twenty to thirty minutes before a meal. The fats can help to reduce your appetite and make you feel satiated more quickly.

Second, if you're not feeling better after a week, this is a sign that your digestive system needs more support. It's best to back off a bit and emphasize the next two sections, which are to incorporate more stocks and stock-based soups as well as lacto-fermented beverages and foods. These in particular have a very calming effect on the entire GI tract. It will also be helpful to supplement with some HCl. Step 3 will discuss supplementation.

But the overwhelming majority of people respond beautifully to eliminating grains and eating good quality fats and protein! This one simple change may be all it takes for your heartburn to slowly fade away if not stop immediately.

## A Word About Nuts, Seeds, and Legumes

One of the big mistakes I see a lot of people make when they go low carb is that they start eating a tremendous amount of nuts and seeds. After all, they're cheap, and they make a great, easily transportable snack. While OK in moderation, consider this:

You're hungry. Like *starving* hungry. What sounds more nourishing? A plate of almonds? Or a big fat juicy steak?

I think there's an innate reason why we crave animal fats more than other fat sources. Besides being more nutrient dense, they are also much more digestible. While nuts and seeds also contain healthy fat and protein, they can be problematic for those with more sensitive systems. Similar to grains, nuts and seeds are best prepared by soaking overnight, which makes them more digestible.

Legumes too need long soaking periods. Furthermore, because they can be high in carbohydrates, legumes can ferment in the stomach and intestines, causing excess gas and bloating. Everyone knows that a dinner of rice and beans can contribute to some embarrassing social situations the next day.

Because commercial versions of nuts, seeds, and legumes rarely go through such a process, it's best to lay off them for the initial two-week period unless you're going to prepare them properly at home. Even then, keep them in moderation for the first month. Part IV will contain some healthy snack ideas to help you find some quick and easy alternatives to nuts and seeds.

## But I'm Hungry All the Time!

This is not uncommon when some transition to a low-carb diet. Years of high-sugar and low-fat and no-fat diets can really whack out your metabolism. High-sugar diets contribute to higher levels of sugar in your blood, which has serious metabolic consequences over the long term. Without healthy fats and protein to balance things out, high-sugar diets also cause low blood sugar, known as hypoglycemia. Low and high blood sugar are often two sides of the same coin, which is eating too much sugar. A vicious cycle can develop in which one constantly craves sugar and carbs. Weight gain, fatigue and, of course, heartburn and digestive problems can result.

Our bodies can be so used to using sugar for energy that there can be a transition period to using fat as energy. As a result, we may experience hunger even when eating more calories. This usually resolves on its own after a few days. If it doesn't, make sure you're not eating zero carbs. That's not the idea here. Your body still needs energy from carbs. This is one of the pitfalls of more extreme low-carb diets, and this is NOT what I want you to do. If you're feeling weak, tired, and hungry, consider adding in some starchier root vegetables. Potatoes, both regular and sweet, would be a good example. They are much easier on the body's digestion than grains. Just don't eat them alone. Enjoy them with fat and protein. This should help balance out the cravings and make you feel more satiated as your body transitions away from a high-sugar diet.

**But I don't know how much fat and protein I should eat!**

Some people are so used to counting calories that they find it strange when I tell them to learn to listen to their body's own hunger signals. If you're a chronic calorie counter, please stop. Eating well should not be a math equation. In fact, most find it liberating when they stop obsessing over calories or counting points or whatever gimmicky approach the latest fad diet is promoting. The idea behind eating more fat and protein is that they will signal satiation more quickly than just eating carbohydrates. You won't need to count calories. Your body will tell you when it's hungry. Again, this may take a few days to a few weeks to level out after years of eating a carbohydrate-based diet, but it will resolve over time.

Have faith in real food!

# 2. The Upper GI – Part II

**Support the pancreas and gallbladder (the pulses on the blender) with beet kvass.**

Beet kvass is a lacto-fermented beverage of Russian origin, and it is truly a digestive powerhouse. According to Sally Fallon in *Nourishing Traditions*:

Beet kvass is "valuable for its medicinal qualities and as a digestive aid. Beets are loaded with nutrients. One glass morning and night is an excellent blood tonic, promotes regularity, aids digestion, alkalizes the blood, cleanses the liver, and is a good treatment for kidney stones and other ailments."[1]

Beet kvass contains three things in particular that will help boost acidity and restore digestive function.

The first is betaine hydrochloride, which helps with the production of stomach acid. Beets are one of the best natural sources, and in fact, they are the most common source for HCl in supplement form. Betaine hydrochloride is also recognized for its role in liver and gallbladder health. An analogy I've frequently heard is that beets are to bile as paint thinner is to paint. In other words, they help promote good bile flow. That's why you will see many liver and gallbladder supplements that contain beet extracts. Beet kvass is therefore an excellent tonic for helping the body digest fats. In particular, it is excellent for those with gallbladder problems or even those without a gallbladder.

The second thing beet kvass contains is enzymes. The lacto-fermentation process increases the enzyme content, and this will help support the pancreas whose job is to add additional digestive enzymes once the food has left the stomach.

So right here we have a drink that will help both the gallbladder and the pancreas. These are the two organs that I made the analogy to the pulse settings on a blender back in Part I. They finish the job in the upper GI so that food is thoroughly digested and prepared for easy absorption in the small intestine.

The third thing beet kvass contains is healthy bacteria as the lacto-fermentation process also increases the probiotic content.

This will help restore a healthy gut flora, reduce fermentation in the gut, and promote overall good digestion.

Beet kvass is a perfect example of why real food is so healing to the body. It not only helps stomach function, it also helps all points further south. It's also a good example of why I prefer to use real food first before trying supplementation.

Best of all, it is SO EASY to make at home. Beet kvass is not something you need to drink in large quantities. It's used more medicinally in small quantities. Take a quarter to a half cup at various intervals throughout the day. Morning and evening are two good times to take it.

Chapter 15 has a simple recipe.

### Troubleshooting

### But I Don't Like Beet Kvass!

Beet kvass has a sour, salty, and sweet flavor that can be a bit shocking to the taste buds the first time you try it. You can dilute it with water if that helps, but most people adjust to it without a problem. Admittedly, I've never quite warmed up to its flavor. I find it strong and somewhat unpleasant but not unpleasant enough that I can't drink it. But if you really can't handle the flavor, there are other lacto-fermented beverages that you can try.

Did you know that many of today's sodas evolved from lacto-fermented beverages? Ginger ale and root beer would be two good examples. Another good option is kombucha, which most find has a very mild flavor. Kombucha also comes from Asia and has been used for thousands of years as a digestive tonic. The good thing about kombucha is that, unlike other lacto-fermented beverages, it is readily available in most health food stores. But it's also easy to make at home. You'll find recipes for both kombucha and ginger ale in the recipes section.

As far as how much ginger ale or kombucha to drink, everyone is different. For those with more chronic digestive issues, sometimes fermented foods can cause some digestive upset. Start slow, watch your symptoms, and gradually increase the amount until you can tolerate about a full glass per day. Some prefer more, some less. Everyone is different.

Regardless which fermented beverage you gravitate towards, try to start incorporating at least one into your daily routine.

## 3. The Middle GI

**Improve nutrient absorption and restore the small intestine lining (the spongy wall) with bone broths.**

Going grain-free, eating good quality fats and protein, and drinking some lacto-fermented beverages will work wonders for restoring proper acidity in your stomach. And as your heartburn and GERD start to fade, so too will other aspects of intestinal distress—gas, bloating, constipation, etc. Again, proper acidity is a domino effect that sets up a chain reaction of events further south.

One thing in particular that can accelerate this process is the use of bone broths, the third pillar of traditional diets. As we've seen, bone broths are prepared by simmering bones in water for long periods of time, which leaches the nutrients out of them. In Part II, I focused on the high mineral content of bone broths.

A good bone broth will contain more than just minerals, though. Meat, skin, bone marrow, cartilage, and tendons attached to a variety of different bones are also part of a good bone stock. Many of these fibrous tissues are composed of a highly dense network of proteins known as collagen. Collagen is only found in animal sources in nature. The proteins in collagen also break down in a good bone broth and reassemble themselves into the strong but pliable tissues in our body such as our joints, skin, and nails. In fact, you may have heard of two such components of collagen, glucosamine and chondroitin sulfates, which are sold as supplements for those with joint problems such as osteoarthritis.

### Gelatin is not just for Jell-O!

An even more familiar component of collagen is gelatin. Gelatin is a waxy substance that forms when broths cool. It's the key ingredient that gives Jell-O its jelly-like consistency. Gelatin has been prized for centuries by cultures around the world for its numerous health benefits, in particular its ability to help ease gastrointestinal discomfort.

Nutritionist Dr. Kaayla Daniel, in her article "Why Broth is Beautiful," discusses the role gelatin played in the medical profession in the first part of the twentieth century. She cites numerous researchers that studied its benefits and doctors that used it therapeutically with patients for an assortment of digestive problems including bacterial infections, inflammation, IBS, and dysbiosis.[2]

In particular, Dr. Daniel quotes the research of Dr. Francis Pottenger, who in 1937 said, "Gelatin may be used in conjunction with almost any diet that the clinician feels is indicated. Its colloidal properties aid the digestion of any foods which cause the patient to suffer from 'sour stomach.'"[3]

"Sour stomach" essentially means heartburn.

Dr. Daniel cites another researcher who in 1872 "found that gelatin improved digestion because of its ability to normalize cases of both hydrochloric acid deficiencies and excesses, and was said to belong in the class of 'peptogenic' substances that favor the flow of gastric juices, thus promoting digestion."[4]

Gelatin also acts as an anti-inflammatory on the gastrointestinal lining. In particular, proline and glycine, the two main amino acids in gelatin, have a profound healing and protective effect.[5]

Gelatin also has hydrophilic properties, meaning it attracts water and helps move food through the digestive system. It is thought that this is another mechanism by which gelatin acts as an anti-inflammatory—it acts as a sort of lubricant in the digestive tract and facilitates the movement of harder to digest foods through the digestive canal.

Hence, gelatin is wonderful for the spongy wall of our intestines as it will nourish and repair the delicate mucosal lining. This will help reverse "leaky gut" by preventing the damaging effects of harder to digest foods and the resulting buildup of bad bacteria (which contributes to dysbiosis and the production of excess gas and pressure).

And the benefits of a good bone broth go far beyond digestion as well. As mentioned previously, chondroitin sulfates and glucosamine are two nutrients that leach out of collagen in bone broths and benefit our joints. Highly popular in supplement form, few people realize that a good broth will supply them in a more absorbable form as well as supply them with so many other beneficial nutrients. Collagen also makes up a large percentage of our skin, hair, and nails.

In my own experience, I can also attest to the calming effect I often feel when I have a good soup with a homemade stock. Almost instantly, I can feel my body relax. And I never sleep better than when I have a nourishing bowl of broth-based soup for dinner. Perhaps it's the calming effect of the minerals. Perhaps it boosts our melatonin levels or eases our cortisol levels or both. I don't know. One study suggests it's the glycine, an amino acid in gelatin that promotes both alertness during the day and restful sleep at night.[6] Whatever the mechanism, many people also report great sleep in conjunction with a good bowl of homemade soup.

## Learn to Make Bone Broths

The bottom line is that it will very helpful to start making bone broths on a regular basis and using them as a base for simple soups and stews. This is especially true if incorporating more fat and protein initially makes you feel heavy or bloated.

If this is the case, for the first few weeks, incorporate bone broth soups liberally. You can have them at any meal, including breakfast; between meals as a digestive tonic; and before bedtime to calm and soothe the nerves. There is no limit to how much and how often you can consume them. Let your symptoms guide you.

## Troubleshooting

### But I've Never Made a Bone Broth!

In the recipe section, you'll find recipes for the three most basic broths. You can also check out my YouTube video for how to make chicken and beef broth: (http://bit.ly/1zTB37E). Half the battle is making them, which is really quite easy. The other half is using them! We're so used to canned soups and bouillon cubes that most Americans have never even made a truly nourishing homemade soup. As proof, check out the soup aisle of any conventional supermarket. The choices are bewildering. Not too long ago I was curious and counted ninety-four varieties of Campbell's soup and seventy-four of Progresso. *All in one aisle.*

If you're not experienced with making homemade soups, don't worry. Soups are so easy to make and can be made into an almost infinite variety of simple, nourishing creations. Better yet, with a little practice, they can be made quickly and without the use of recipes.

All you need to learn is a few basic steps. Once memorized, the world is your soup pot!

### 3 Steps to Broth-Based Soups

Here's the basic formula:

- Step 1. Sauté hard vegetables in butter and/or good quality olive oil for 5–10 minutes.
- Step 2. Add stock, bring to a boil, and simmer another 5–10 minutes.
- Step 3. Add soft vegetables and soft meat and cook another 5–10 minutes and season to taste.

In step one, "hard vegetables" means any vegetables that need a little heat to soften. Those are usually your root vegetables like onions, garlic, carrots, celery, and leeks. This initial heating will also soften the sharper flavors of these vegetables and add more depth and complexity to your soup.

Step two is pretty straightforward. Heat up the stock and simmer. You can bring out more flavor in these vegetables by simmering them a lot longer than 5–10 minutes, but only if you have the time. I rarely do. If you're really in a rush, you can even combine steps one and two. That is, add the vegetables to the stock and heat them together.

In step three, "soft vegetables" means any vegetables that only need a little heat to soften. For the most part, that's greens. I always add them at the end. But I like most of my veggies fairly crisp, even in my soups, so I'll also add things like Brussels sprouts or string beans towards the end as well. If you want to cook them longer, by all means, go for it.

"Soft meats" mean things like chicken, fish, and shellfish. They cook through fairly quickly. Harder cuts of meat like tougher cuts of red meat need a longer cooking time to break down the fibers and gelatinous connective tissue and are better for stews.

Now I know some hard-core chefs out there might roll their eyes at this basic three-step process. I know this summary is not exactly fine French cooking. But I'm not interested in the finer points of cooking. And you know what? Neither are the majority of stressed-out, overworked parents, working folks, students, and, well, basically everyone I know who lives in America.

That's why I like to say that to eat well, you don't need to be a chef, but you do need to be a cook. We're not trying to be Julia Child here. We are trying to be realistic. Nevertheless, to truly stop heartburn and GERD, we do need to spend a *little* more time in our kitchens. Learning to make your own soups can go a long way towards reducing the amount of time you spend in your kitchen preparing meals from scratch.

## 4. The lower GI

**Restore the biodiversity of the intestines (the rainforest) with fermented foods.**

Fermented foods are the final pillar of real food, and they are a digestive powerhouse in every sense from the top of our digestive system all the way down.

Let's start right where heartburn occurs, in the stomach and esophagus. Years of poor diet, low stomach acid, and bacterial overgrowth can inflame and aggravate the lining of the esophagus and the stomach. Heartburn as well as gastritis, *H. pylori*, and ulcers are all connected by inflammation in that delicate lining. The bacteria in fermented foods have been shown to have an anti-inflammatory effect on the lining of the stomach.[7]

Fermented foods are also rich in enzymes, which help us break down and digest our food properly. Our body's production of enzymes naturally decreases as we age. Years of heartburn and low stomach acid can also compromise the pancreas' ability to produce digestive enzymes. Fermented foods can help ease the burden on the pancreas by providing a rich supply in the diet. Adding lacto-fermented beverages will also support this process.

Fermented foods are also rich in healthy bacteria, probably their most widely known benefit. They will help restore the rich diversity of bacterial life in the intestines, which I compared to the Amazon rainforest back in Chapter 10.

### Probiotics are not Just Supplements

These good bacteria are also called "probiotics," and millions now take them in supplement form. But it's much better to get them from real fermented foods, which also deliver actual *nutrients* in addition to probiotics. And keep in mind that probiotic supplements are *proprietary* strains. That means they are formulated in laboratories by companies so they can be patented and then sold for profit. Not that there is anything wrong with that. Many companies put out effective probiotic supplements. Dozens of studies using probiotic therapy show benefits in treating a wide variety of digestive issues. However, few studies have ever been done with actual fermented foods. Why? Because you can't patent sauerkraut. Or kimchi. Or any food for that matter.

According to Dr. Mercola on his website, one serving of fermented vegetables has 100 times more beneficial bacteria than an entire bottle of a high-potency probiotic product![8]

And let's not forget that fermented foods are an integral part of the diet of every traditional culture on this planet. They have been around as long as humans have been around. It is only recently, with the advent of refrigeration and processed foods, that many industrialized societies have stopped using traditionally fermented foods.

While we can't deny the benefits of probiotic supplementation, over the long term, I trust the thousands of years of fermented foods in the human diet more than laboratory formulations. Give me fermented foods over supplements any day. They are much tastier, too.

Most health food stores carry at least a few good brands of fermented dairy, sauerkraut, and pickles. For fermented vegetables, check the labels, and make sure you don't see vinegar or preservatives. You may also find things like kimchi, pickled beets, and ginger carrots. The heartburn resources page on my website also lists some quality companies that you can order from online. (http://fearlesseating.net/heartburn-book-resources)

For fermented dairy, seek out raw milk cheese if you can. Other forms of fermented dairy such as yogurt and kefir will be pasteurized, but good quality can still be had. Make sure you see "contains live cultures" on the label. That means the company added good bacteria *after* pasteurization. And of course, find companies that source milk from grass-fed cows.

## Learn to Make Fermented Vegetables at Home

Ultimately though, it's a lot more rewarding and cost efficient to make fermented vegetables at home. Best of all, it's so easy! The recipe section will include recipes for making sauerkraut, pickles, and kimchi.

## Troubleshooting

## But I'm Afraid I'll Sicken Myself!

I hear this a lot when folks start to experiment with fermenting foods at home. Many are hesitant to keep foods out at room temperature, which is necessary in the initial stages of fermentation. I have been lucky enough to see Sandor Katz, fermentation guru and author of *Wild Fermentation* and *The Art of Fermentation,* speak on a few occasions. He likes to point out that in his travels and experiences, he has never met one person who has ever become sick from fermenting foods at home.

According to Fred Breidt, a microbiologist with the USDA:

"With fermented products there is no safety concern. I can flat out say that. The reason is the lactic acid bacteria that carry out the fermentation are the world's best killer of other bacteria."

Breidt goes on to say that, regarding fermented vegetables, "there are no known documented cases of food-borne illness."

Remember, fermentation is a process by which bad bacteria cannot grow. So don't stress it! You'll be fine.

## But I Don't Like the Taste of Fermented Foods!

I come across this all the time. Most kids of my generation grew up without ever consuming any real fermented foods. Yogurt is the perfect example. Whole milk PLAIN yogurt has a natural sweetness due to the sugars present in milk. It is mildly and pleasantly sweet. But most kids find it tasteless if there's no added sugar. They're used to commercial, fruit-flavored yogurts, which of course are sweetened to death with sugar, high-fructose corn syrup, and natural flavors more than any fruit.

Because our taste buds are so addicted to sugar these days, traditionally fermented foods can be a bit shocking to the taste buds. And to the nose as well! I'll often include some of my homemade fermented vegetables when I'm packing a lunch or dinner. The reaction is pretty predictable. "Ewww, what's that smell?" is what almost everyone says whenever I pop open a jar of my homemade sauerkraut or kimchi.

But it never ceases to amaze me how quickly our taste buds adjust to real foods. Properly fermented foods are a perfect example. And they are not so much an acquired taste as they are a reacquired taste. I say "reacquired" because, traditionally speaking, they were a part of all native diets.

If you don't like their taste, be patient and go slow. Start with the more familiar items like pickles or yogurt. Over time, I'm confident you will start to naturally crave and enjoy them.

## But Fermented Foods Make My Digestion Worse!

Though rare, some can experience problems when first introducing fermented foods. This is usually a sign of dysbiosis, which means an imbalance of good to bad bacteria in the gut.

Eating a low-carb diet while introducing fermented foods can cause what's known as a "die-off" reaction. This means that the healthy bacteria are killing off the bad bacteria, which can cause unpleasant symptoms such as fatigue, muscle aches, headaches, skin rashes, and further GI problems such as excess gas, bloating, diarrhea, or constipation.

If this happens, go slow. Start with just a teaspoon of some sauerkraut juice and see how you do. Slowly increase the amount until you're having a very small amount of actual sauerkraut or perhaps a bite of a pickle. Slowly increase the amount until you can tolerate it. Fermented vegetables are not meant to be consumed in large quantities. A quarter to a half cup as a side dish is all that's needed under normal conditions.

There's also the issue of the fiber in not only fermented vegetables but also fiber-rich foods such as fruits, vegetables, grains (another good reason to remove them), legumes, and nuts. Fiber does not break down in our digestive tract but helps move food through it. However, fiber-rich foods can be irritating to the digestive lining if it's been compromised. If this is the case for you, gravitate towards fermented beverages and fermented dairy for the time being. Include lots of bone broth-based soups as well.

## 5. Use raw milk as an antacid

Did you know that raw milk was actually used as a traditional remedy for heartburn?

Though this knowledge has been lost to most of us who grew up with low-fat, pasteurized milk from CAFOs, it still lives on in those with a connection to a more agrarian-based America. Baby boomers and those who grew up before WWII can probably tell you of their mothers, grandmothers, and maybe great-grandmothers who used raw milk as a tonic to settle all sorts of digestive disturbances including, of course, heartburn, or as they might have called it back in the day, "sour stomach" or "agita" or maybe just "indigestion."

Even the medical profession prescribed raw milk as a digestive tonic back in the day. In fact, raw milk fasts were common in the early decades of the 1900s as a treatment for reversing serious health problems. In particular, The Mayo Foundation, the precursor to the Mayo Clinic, used to use raw milk fasts to treat their patients.[9]

Even today, anecdotal evidence is widespread. You'll see tons of testimonials online of the heartburn-quelching effects of drinking milk. The calcium in milk buffers stomach acid similarly to antacids like TUMS.

**TUMS vs. Raw Milk**

The active ingredient in TUMS is calcium carbonate, which works well to neutralize stomach acid. But let's take a look at what else is in TUMS. Here's the ingredients label for the Ultra Strength 1000 Assorted Fruit Flavored TUMS:

Sucrose, calcium carbonate, corn starch, talc, mineral oil, natural and artificial flavors, adipic acid, sodium polyphosphate, red 40 lake, yellow 6 lake, yellow 5 (tartrazine) lake, blue 1 lake.

In case the Assorted Fruit flavor doesn't float your boat, TUMS also has Berry Fusion, Assorted Berries, Tropical Fruit, and Orange Cream flavors also jam-packed with sugar and chemicals.

With raw milk, you will not get any of the chemicals listed above. Instead, you'll get calcium and other minerals (in a highly absorbable form), vitamins A, D, E, K, C, B, conjugated linoleic acid, omega-3s, amino acids, enzymes, and healthy bacteria.

Which would you choose?

There could well be other factors both separate and complementary that make raw milk such an excellent digestive tonic. Some say the fats in milk help to soothe and coat the esophageal and gastric lining. It's almost impossible to know how all the nutrients in whole foods, both known and unknown, work in the body.

But who cares how it works, right? The point is that if it does work for you, then go with it. You'll not only be helping your symptoms, you'll also be adding another traditional, nutrient-dense food to your diet that has benefits well beyond just easing heartburn symptoms.

There are no absolutes when it comes to drinking raw milk, but here's what I recommend.

First, use raw milk as you would an antacid. When heartburn hits after a meal, drink a glass of raw milk. See how it makes you feel. If it settles things down, well then, great! But don't overdo it, initially. Raw milk is still high in carbohydrates and could possibly contribute to some bacterial imbalances and fermentation in the gut. The healthy fats and protein in milk should buffer that effect, but everyone is different. If you do notice some digestive disturbances, then back off and let the other real food pillars work first. You can try raw milk later on, but don't feel like you have to if everything else is proceeding well.

Second, if your body responds well to raw milk, you can start to incorporate it more often. This will be especially helpful if initially incorporating more fat and protein makes you feel bloated. Similar to bone broths, raw milk presents a wide variety of nutrients in easily absorbable form.

**Troubleshooting**

**But I Can't Get Raw Milk**

Unfortunately, raw milk is difficult to access in most states. It's either illegal or you need to pick it up from the farm or you need to be part of a cow-share program. Again, please see www.realmilk.com for a list of raw milk dairies by state.

If you can't get raw milk or perhaps you're just not willing to try it, that's OK too. Raw milk is not absolutely essential to your success. I've included it here as something to help relieve symptoms as you work the other real food pillars. Part III will have a few supplements you can try as well.

## But I'm Lactose Intolerant!

Milk is one of those foods that people have vastly different experiences with, even with fermented dairy. As the expression goes, "one man's meat is another man's poison." Some thrive on it. Some do not. If dairy makes you feel heavy, bloated, gassy, or mucousy, or it aggravates any other symptoms, then just leave it out. Or you may already be diagnosed with a sensitivity such as lactose intolerance. Interestingly, though anecdotal, some with lactose intolerance report they are able to drink raw milk without a problem.[10] I've had many people tell me the exact same thing. Many believe this is due to the enzymes and perhaps other undamaged nutrients present that make it less problematic than pasteurized milk.

Regardless, if you've never tried raw milk, I would highly recommend it as something to experiment with.

## To Supplement or Not to Supplement

I find it hard to imagine that Step 1 and 2, if applied diligently, will not bring about a dramatic improvement in your symptoms.

Nevertheless, if you've experienced long-term GERD with long-term associated health problems, some supplementation can really help.

But ONLY proceed with Step 3 if your symptoms are not improving. This is why I've spent so much time educating you about real food first—this is often all it takes! I do the same thing with private clients. I set them up with dietary changes and then WAIT for two weeks to see if supplementation is needed. If after two weeks things have not progressed significantly, then I'll consider some supplemental support.

# 13

## How to Navigate the Wild West

**S**tep #3 - Soothe and repair with supplementation for the last two weeks *but only if necessary.*

### An Overview of Supplements

The supplement industry today is akin to the Wild West. There is very little regulation, and companies can get away with very deceptive and misleading health claims and labels. As such, not all supplements are created equal and there are many more poor quality brands than good ones. For example, most supplements sold in pharmacies and big-box grocery stores are very poorly made. That is why they are usually cheaper in those places. Most of those supplements contain synthetic minerals and vitamins that are made in a laboratory from non-food ingredients such as petroleum. Others extract isolates of vitamins, which are not whole vitamins. For example, you'll frequently see vitamin C labeled "Vitamin C (as ascorbic acid)." Ascorbic acid is a component of vitamin C but not true vitamin C. Our body does not use isolates the same way it uses whole foods. Some suggest they can even be toxic. Even in health food stores, a brief tour around the supplement section yields a bewildering array of choices and health claims.

When it comes to heartburn and GERD, there are also a wide spectrum of supplements and herbs that may help. Not all supplements work for everyone so it can take some trial and error to find what works for you. This can be somewhat overwhelming.

Because I trust food more than supplements, I've chosen to make Step 3 as simple as possible. For the upper GI tract, I will discuss two different supplements you can try. For the middle and lower GI tract, I recommend just ONE. That's it. The products I recommend are listed on the <u>heartburn resources page</u> on my website. Of course, there are dozens more that could be discussed but to go down that road opens up a Pandora's box of talking about more and more supplements.

Still, I understand that everyone is different and not everyone responds the same to all supplements. After I discuss the ones I recommend, I will briefly mention or just list additional herbs and supplements that are also known to help.

If the supplements I recommend don't work well for you and/or you react to them negatively, I would highly recommend that you work with a knowledgeable practitioner to find ones that do. A word of advice though—if that practitioner is sending you away with a bag load of supplements, be suspicious. Find someone who stresses real food and lifestyle changes before supplementation.

Also, there are contraindications for many supplements including the ones I recommend. Consult with your physician about potential side effects and drug interactions. If you experience any sort of negative side effect with any supplements, STOP taking them.

## Supplement From North to South

We've seen how digestion is supposed to work going from north to south and how it can go wrong. We've seen how real food will start to correct heartburn going from north to south. And finally, *for the last time* (I promise), we will see how supplementation works going north to south, because supplementing works the same way! Correct the acidity in the stomach and all points further south start to correct as well.

## Upper GI Option #1: Turn the blender UP with HCl!

If you have a deficiency in vitamin D, what do you do? You take vitamin D. A deficiency in B12? Take B12. Deficiency in minerals? Supplement with minerals.

Hydrochloric acid is no different. You can literally take HCl in capsule form. You can find HCl in the supplement section of almost any health food store. The most common form you'll find is Betaine HCl. Make sure it also contains pepsin, the protein-digesting enzyme, which works synergistically with HCl. Most brands contain both. Some will also contain pancreatic enzymes and perhaps a few other nutrients known for boosting digestive function, such as vitamin C.

Supplementing with HCl tends to freak people out when they haven't first understood the proper physiology of how acid works in the body. But now that you know that heartburn and GERD are not caused by too much but rather too little acid and that HCl occurs naturally in your stomach, hopefully, you're not too weirded out by this.

Adding HCl will help to boost the blender speed of your stomach so you can start properly digesting your food. Truth be told, I don't love asking people to try HCl. It can be a bit tricky to dose. It's not as simple as just taking fish oil or a multivitamin. The reason is that some people need more than others. If your blender speed has gone from high to medium high, you might only need a little. But if your blender is on low (hypochlorhydria) or is even barely working (achlorhydria), you're going to need a lot more.

You'll need to do an HCl challenge test on yourself, which can help you determine how much you need.

But before I explain that, you should know that, although supplementing with HCl is safe for most people, there are some risks. Dr. Jonathan Wright in *Why Stomach Acid is Good for You* explains:

"People that are 'high risk' shouldn't take Betaine HCl without supervision. You're high risk if you're consuming any anti-inflammatory medicines. Examples of those are corticosteroids, aspirin, Indocin, ibuprofen (Motrin, Advil) or other

NSAIDs. These drugs can damage the GI lining and supplementing with HCl could aggravate it, increasing the risks of bleeding or ulcer."[1]

It really is a good idea to find an experienced practitioner to help you with using HCl. Unfortunately, there is no established way to dose it, and some practitioners have different approaches than others. It can take a bit of trial and error to figure it out. My recommendation and the way I go about it with clients is to go very gently and very slowly.

**HCl Challenge Test**

1. Sit down to a normal meal with some protein.
2. Begin with several bites of food and take one capsule. Continue to eat normally. Do this at each meal on Day 1. I start each client out at 300mg. Many brands include quite a bit more in each capsule, some as much as 650 mg. That's OK, but try to find the smallest starting dose possible.
3. Pay attention to any changes you may feel. In particular, what you're looking for is a warming sensation in your stomach.
4. If no warming sensation is felt on Day 1, increase the dosage by one tablet to a total of two at each meal on Day 2. Increase the dosage by one tablet each day until a warming sensation is reached. So if no warming sensation is felt at one tablet per meal on Day 1, increase to two tablets each meal on Day 2, three on Day 3, four on Day 4, and so on and so forth.
5. Once a warming sensation is reached, back off to the dosage where there was no warming sensation. So if the warming sensation happens with four tablets, your individual dose is 3 tablets.
6. Once you find your individual dosage, take all the tablets together *in the middle or towards the end* of each of your three main meals. If you forget, you can still take them a half hour or so after a meal. There's no exact science to when to take HCl, but most agree that

somewhere between the middle and just after the meal is the best time. You may also have to adjust the dosage, depending on the size of the meal. Lighter meals may require slightly fewer tablets.

7. If no warming sensation is felt after a week of supplementing, do not be alarmed! This is quite common. Dr. Wright has found that, on average, most people need between five to seven 650mg tablets, which works out to around 3000–4500 mg per meal. However, he notes that many will need over 5000 mg per meal for the proper support. That's about ten 500 mg tablets per meal. That may sound excessive, but it is not uncommon. When I was having digestive problems years ago, I was taking about 5000 mg per meal. Over time, I was able to take less and less. Unless you're taking any of the medications listed above, HCl supplementation is very safe.

8. The purpose of HCl supplementation is to encourage your body to boost its own production of stomach acid. Ideally, you should be able to lessen your dose over time. So if you're taking six tablets with each meal, in several weeks you may find you experience a warming sensation with the six tablets. That means it's time to reduce your dosage to five tablets. Simply keep reducing your dosage over time until it is no longer needed. Your body can now produce HCl on its own.

If you experience intense burning and discomfort after one tablet of HCl capsule, stop. The warming sensation you're looking for should not be painful. This is a sign that your stomach lining is compromised and cannot handle HCl yet. Though rare, this can happen in those with chronic inflammation conditions in the stomach lining such as gastritis, *H. pylori*, and ulcers. You'll have to work with Steps 1 and 2 for a longer period. How long? I'd recommend waiting a full month before trying HCl again. You can also try the very common folk remedy of taking some apple cider vinegar.

**Upper GI Option #2: Apple cider vinegar**

Remember Sarah from the Introduction, the woman who wrote me the apology email? If you recall, she mentioned experimenting with taking some acid in lieu of her Nexium. The acid she described taking was actually not HCl. It was vinegar. In the second part of her email, she shared with me a post she wrote on an online message board.

She wrote:

*"I took Nexium for around ten years, and was taking it daily up until recently, when I started having heartburn in spite of it. I decided to investigate the competing theory of the cause of heartburn and acid reflux, namely that it is caused by not enough acid, not by too much acid. My decision was inspired by the logic of the situation: If I was taking Nexium, which supposedly reduced my stomach acid to nearly zero, how, then, could my heartburn be caused by too much acid?*

*So, while actually experiencing heartburn, I took a tablespoon of a 50-50 mix of balsamic vinegar and honey. The heartburn went away in about fifteen minutes. Later in the day, when I got heartburn again, I took some more of the mix, which again quieted my symptoms. Starting that day, I began to increase the interval between Nexium doses, from 24 hours between pills to 25, then 26, etc.*

*At the same time, I took a tablespoon of the honey/vinegar mix at each meal (or more if I felt symptoms) and at each snack, and whenever I had either reflux, heartburn or roiling of the stomach. For the first few days, I felt like I was guzzling the stuff, but I persevered. I was very comfortable and able to eat normally. By the time I got to a 36-hour interval, I started losing track of the process of tapering the Nexium off, and just stopped taking it. Now, two weeks since my last Nexium pill, I feel very well. I have also started taking probiotics… If I could swallow pills easily, which I cannot, I would prefer to take the Betaine HCl pills, just for the convenience… I am thinking about trying to take straight balsamic vinegar, but haven't worked up the courage."*

I'm not sure why Sarah chose balsamic vinegar over apple cider vinegar (ACV) as ACV is more commonly used as a heartburn remedy. But the idea is the same for both. Vinegar is highly acidic (but not as potent as taking HCl in pill form), and the idea is similar to taking HCl in that it gives your stomach a digestive boost. You can start by trying ACV in lieu of HCl if you're hesitant to try HCl.

Mix one to two teaspoons of ACV in water and take it just *before* meals. Some also add a little juice or honey (like Sarah did) to help dilute its strong taste, though I would recommend trying to get it down without the added sugar. If you experience an uncomfortable burn similar to taking one tablet of HCl, then stop taking it. You'll need to work with Steps 1 and 2.

## How to Stop Acid-Blocking Medications

Sarah's description of weaning herself off the acid-blocking medication may not work for everyone. Remember, there are two types of acid-reflux medications: acid-neutralizers and acid-blockers. It is not difficult to stop taking the acid-neutralizers—TUMS, Rolaids, Mylanta, Alka Seltzer, etc. The 3-Step Plan should dramatically reduce your dependency on them. It's getting off the acid-blockers, in particular the proton pump inhibitors—Prilosec, Nexium, Prevacid, etc.—that can be tricky, especially if you've been taking them for a long period.

Many experience a rebound effect when they attempt to stop taking PPIs, which can lead to a worsening of symptoms. This rebound effect is not uncommon and is known as "rebound acid hypersecretion." Because acid secretion is shut down by PPIs, the stomach can start over-producing acid once the PPI therapy is stopped. In some cases, this can last for weeks or even months.

A 2009 study was performed in the journal *Gastroenterology* on *healthy* individuals without any prior symptoms of heartburn. They took PPIs for eight weeks. Over 40% of the study participants reported *increased symptoms of heartburn* **after** *they stopped taking the PPIs.*[2]

This is why so many become dependent on them. If they stop, the reflux comes right back with a vengeance. That being said, I've had many clients stop taking them *without* rebound acid hypersecretion. But I *never* instruct them to do this. It's not my place to tell my clients to stop taking medications. I simply inform and educate them so they can make their own decisions. Many will discuss stopping their medications with their doctor but many won't because they know they'll be dismissed.

But let's give some doctors the benefit of the doubt. They're overworked and don't have much time to do their own research. Most are not aware of the long-term risks of taking acid-blockers. Share with him/her the study, "Overutilization of proton pump inhibitors: what the clinician needs to know," published in *Therapeutic Advances in Gastroenterology.*

The conclusion of the study stated:

*"PPIs have been linked via retrospective studies to increased risk of enteric infections including Clostridium difficile–associated diarrhea, community-acquired pneumonia, bone fracture, nutritional deficiencies, and interference with metabolism of antiplatelet agents. Reducing inappropriate prescribing of PPIs in the inpatient and outpatient settings can minimize potential for adverse events, and foster controllable cost expenditure."*

You can print it out here:
http://www.ncbi.nlm.nih.gov/pubmed/22778788

To stop taking your PPIs, you'll have to make a judgment call whether to go cold turkey or to wean off them more slowly. For mild to moderate cases, I'd recommend going cold turkey. *But make sure you've made the dietary changes in Steps 1 and 2 for at least a few weeks.* When you feel ready, stop taking them. If the acid reflux comes back after a few days but you feel it's manageable, take the HCl or ACV with meals as described above. Continue to work with the dietary changes and the supplements (including the ones listed below for the middle and lower GI) as the acid reflux decreases over time.

However, if after going cold turkey the acid reflux comes raging back, you'll have to wean off them more slowly. It's good to find a knowledgeable practitioner to help you with this. Naturopathic doctors (NDs), Nutritional Therapists (NTPs), many chiropractors, and even some medical doctors employing natural approaches can help.

Here's what I recommend (and by all means, write this down and share it with your practitioner):

1. Be sure the dietary changes discussed in Steps 1 and 2 are firmly in place for at least a few weeks.
2. When you feel ready, start reducing the dosage of your acid-blocker. So if you're taking 40 mg once a day, start taking 20 mg instead.
3. Start increasing the intervals at which you take your daily dose. Go from once every 24 hours to once every 36 hours. If all goes well, then start taking it every other day. If that proceeds well, take it every third day. And so on and so forth until you stop taking them altogether.
4. All the while, work with the HCl or ACV to boost your digestive capacity. If an episode hits, try taking some ACV or raw milk in the middle of it. The juice of fermented beverages can also help knock out an episode—sauerkraut or pickle juice work well for many.
5. Take the supplements for the middle and lower GI (cod liver oil and probiotics) as described below.

Weaning off PPIs can take some trial and error. Some of the other supplements mentioned below may also help. It's rarely a smooth process so don't get discouraged if your acid reflux comes back at times. If episodes are lessening in their intensity and frequency, know that you're on the right track.

## Other Upper GI Supplement Options

### Digestive Enzymes

Personally, I prefer to use HCl over digestive enzymes because once the HCl is being produced adequately, so too will digestive enzymes, at least in theory. I also use an HCl product that contains a little pancreatin, a mixture of pancreatic enzymes. It is common to find HCl and enzymes together in supplement form. Still, some may do better than others with digestive enzymes, especially if HCl causes irritation. If so, take 1-2 capsules with each meal as a digestive boost. And don't forget those enzyme-rich fermented beverages and foods!

### Bitters

I don't have much experience with bitters as I've found that almost everyone starts experiencing relief with dietary changes and then HCl. Nevertheless, bitters are commonly used for heartburn and are mentioned here as a possible alternative to HCl if there is gastric inflammation.

Bitters are just that, bitter. The idea is that bitter substances promote the production of HCl. They usually come in liquid form from herbs and are highly concentrated so that only a drop or two is needed either dissolved in a little water or placed right on the tongue. You'll find them in most health food stores. Dandelion, gentian, and wormwood are a few examples of common bitters.

### Other Herbs and Supplements That May Help.

Deglycyrrhizinated licorice(DGL), L-glutamine, ginger, turmeric, vitamin A, vitamin C, and herbal teas such as chamomile and ginger may also help.

### The Middle GI: Repair the spongy wall with Fermented Cod Liver Oil.

The demand for fish oil today can easily be seen in the supplement aisle of any store. There are hundreds of companies manufacturing fish oil. Except for one, they all extract the oils from fish using high-tech methods that can remove the oils quickly and efficiently. However, all of these methods damage the fragile nutrients to some degree.

Have you ever wondered how people extracted the oils from fish before industrialization?

Simple. They let the fish sit in barrels and, over time, the oils would naturally leach out and rise to the surface. This process of fermentation has the added benefit of preserving and enhancing the nutrient content. Cod liver oil in particular is a good source of anti-inflammatory omega-3 essential fatty acids and also a great source of vitamins A and D, both of which play dozens of important roles in the body, including promoting a healthy gut lining.

According to Dr. Natasha Campbell McBride in *Gut and Psychology Syndrome*:

"In fact, gut disease is one of the symptoms of vitamin A deficiency because the gut lining is one of the most active sites of cell production, growth, and differentiation. Neither of these processes can happen properly without a good supply of vitamin A. Leaky gut and malabsorption are the typical results of vitamin A deficiency." [3]

Studies also show vitamin D plays a role in the integrity of the gut lining.[4]

Green Pasture is the one company, as of now, that is producing cod liver oil by the traditional fermentation method in the United States. Because this traditional method takes *time*, you won't find it on the shelves of popular health food stores. They simply can't produce it fast enough to supply large retail outlets like Whole Foods. You can find Green Pasture on the heartburnresources page on my website.

These are the dosing recommendations from the Weston Price Foundation:

– Children, age 3 months to 12 years – 1/2 tsp
– Adults – 1 tsp
– Pregnant or nursing women – 2 tsp

If you have experienced chronic GERD for an extended period, and if after two weeks you have not seen a significant improvement in your symptoms, I would recommend taking two to three teaspoons of fermented cod liver for a few months as an additional boost. After that, take one teaspoon per day.

Beyond heartburn, fermented cod liver oil can be taken for overall general health. I use it in lieu of multivitamins as it contains the fat-soluble vitamins in absorbable form that so many people are deficient in, in particular A, D, E, and K2.

For a more extensive look into cod liver oil manufacturing:
http://www.westonaprice.org/health-topics/update-on-cod-liver-oil-manufacture/

## Fermented Cod Liver Oil Alternatives

There are many supplements that can help restore the lining of both the stomach and intestines. Two of the more common ones are deglycyrrhizinated licorice (DGL) and L-glutamine. DGL comes from licorice root and L-glutamine is an amino acid. Both have been shown to promote the integrity of the intestinal lining. Aloe vera juice is another supplement that has been shown to have anti-inflammatory effects on the digestive lining.

## The Lower GI: Repopulate the Rainforest with Probiotics.

Though probiotics in food form is the ideal, taking a probiotic supplement can certainly support the process of reestablishing a healthy gut flora.

As with all supplements, there are dozens, if not hundreds, of companies to choose from. Here is what you should look for in a good probiotic supplement:

1. A wide spectrum of bacterial species. Remember, there are hundreds of different species that populate your gut. A good probiotic will contain as many as possible. You should see several species in the Lactobacillus and Bifidobacteria families like *Lactobacillus acidophilus* ( *L. acidophilus*) and *Bifidobacteria bifidum* (*B. bifidum*). A good probiotic will contain others as well. A good rule of thumb is to find a product with at least seven or eight different species.

2. Make sure you see "colony forming units" (CFUs) listed in the billions. Take approximately 8 to 15 billion CFUs per capsule. At two capsules per day that equates to 16 to 30 billion CFUs per day. There is a wide variety of opinion on this, but most practitioners suggest this range for therapeutic purposes.

3. CFUs that are *guaranteed* at the time of expiration on the bottle. The CFUs should be guaranteed to be alive well after the time you purchase the probiotic. Many companies will print the CFUs at the time of manufacture, which does not guarantee they will be alive by the time they get to the supermarket shelves.

Most probiotics require refrigeration. Check each product for specific instructions for storage.

Also, some probiotics come with an enteric coating that is designed to withstand the acidity of the stomach. Personally, I don't worry about this, as humans have been consuming probiotics for thousands of years. Furthermore, the stomach needs beneficial bacteria as well.

Take one capsule on an empty stomach in the morning and evening. If those times don't suit you, other times between meals are fine. To start, I would take them for at least a month. If things are going well after a month, your symptoms are gone, and you're regularly consuming fermented foods, then it is fine to discontinue them. If things are not completely resolved but improving, then continue to take the probiotics for as long as you feel they are benefitting you.

# Part IV

Putting It All Together

# 14

# Meal Planning Tips

It's insane that it's almost impossible to find healthy food when you leave your house. A "food desert" is a relatively new term that describes an area with little access to real food. Though it's mostly used in the context of low-income urban areas, I think it describes many suburban areas as well. Big box supermarkets, gas stations, malls, fast-food establishments, airports, and sporting arenas offer almost nothing in the way of sustainably grown, nutrient-dense food. Even schools and hospitals have become co-opted by industrialized food.

Sometimes your hands will be tied and there's nothing you can do. Don't stress it. But for the most part, you do need to start getting comfortable with cooking more and preparing meals at home because continually eating out, ordering out, using the microwave, and eating frozen meals and quick-prepared food out of cans and boxes is a slow but sure route to poor health. It may be what got you into trouble in the first place.

There is no way around it; eating well takes planning. The most important thing to understand is that **planning is the key to your success**. But it is well worth the time and effort.

The sections that follow include recipes, meal ideas, and two very simple grain-free meal plans to help you put the 3-Step Plan into action.

## Recipes

Please be sure to become familiar with the recipes for fermented foods, bone stocks, and soups. They are so important for all the reasons we've discussed. Start simple. Purchase or make one fermented vegetable. Choose the fermented beverage that most appeals to you and try it out. You can sample some kombucha in your local health food store to start. Next, make one of the stocks and make one soup from it.

I've also decided to include some recipes for making some simple homemade salad dressings, as store-bought versions are an absolute horror show of chemicals. Salads with a good protein are quick and easy to prepare at home. They will also be very helpful if you're a working person going through the grain-free stage.

Finally, you'll see two simple recipes for grain-free breads. These will help those of you that really miss bread and/or experience intense carb cravings in the grain-free stage.

## Meal Ideas Instead of Meal Plans

After the recipes, you'll see a list of ideas for breakfast, lunch, dinner, and snacks. These are by no means exhaustive lists. They are just meant to get you going in the right direction and to help stimulate ideas for a variety of meals. Use whatever works for you.

Personally, I *much prefer* meal ideas to meal plans. In fact, I have a confession. I *hate* meal plans. I really do. I look at most meal plans I see on the internet and shake my head in disbelief or just laugh. They are just so UNREALISTIC. Most have 21 different meals for each of the three meals of the week. You'd better either be retired or independently wealthy and not working to make most of these meal plans doable. Then, of course, there are different personal tastes, different work and family schedules, and the myriad food sensitivities these days that make so many meal plans difficult to follow.

That being said, I understand that initially some written meal plans can be helpful, especially in the grain-free stage. So I've included two that you can work from to get you going.

**Meal Planning Tips**

Instead of highly specific meal plans, use the meal ideas presented here to develop your own meal plans. Or maybe you're not a meal plan sort of person who needs to map out the whole week. That's fine too. Regardless, some degree of planning is helpful. Here are five simple tips:

**1. Cook one to two meals each week in bulk.**

There is no need to cook every meal from scratch. You'll drive yourself absolutely crazy. Cook one to two meals in bulk each week that you will reuse throughout the week. I try to cook a big pot of soup each week. There's nothing better than coming home when you're tired and having dinner ready via a simple reheat. Soups and stews are ideal for cooking in bulk. Roasts, whole chickens, hams, and other larger cuts of meat are great for cooking in bulk as well. Freeze whatever you won't use throughout the week.

**2. Always have versatile ingredients on hand for quick and easy meals.**

To me, there's nothing that fits this better than eggs. As Jessica Prentice says in her book *Full Moon Feast*, "Eggs are the original fast food."

You can prepare them in dozens of different ways. Endless combinations of veggies and healthy starches can keep egg dishes from getting boring. And they work just as well for lunch and dinner as they do for breakfast. You can never go wrong with eggs.

You could say the same for salads and soups as well. So versatile, so easy, and they work for each of your three main meals.

### 3. Have good resources on hand.

This is important when you feel stuck. These are my three personal favorites:

Google. I always have my computer on in my kitchen and will search the internet for recipe ideas when needed. There are dozens of great websites. Print out recipes for future use when you come across good ones. Create a binder to organize them. Just remember that most recipe websites are not about using real food. For example, most sites will use poor-quality vegetable oils or pre-packaged items like bouillon cubes. Always substitute real food ingredients as much as possible.

*Nourishing Traditions* by Sally Fallon. Please purchase this wonderful cookbook and educational resource. You will use it for decades to come. It brings the principles of traditional diets into modern life with easy-to-use recipes. You'll find it on the heartburn resources page on my website:
(http://www.fearlesseating.net/heartburn-book-resources)

Nourished Kitchen. This is a fantastic online resource with hundreds of great traditional food recipes. There will be no need to substitute any ingredients here. www.nourishedkitchen.com

### 4. Try one new recipe each week.

Routine is good. Boredom is not. It's easy to get into ruts where we make the same things over and over and over. If cooking is foreign to you, that's OK. Start with a few simple recipes and don't overwhelm yourself. Weekends are good times to experiment with new ideas. Use the above resources to generate new ideas when you get stuck.

### 5. Be fearless and have fun.

"Learn how to cook. Try new recipes, learn from your mistakes, be fearless, and have fun." - Julia Child

I understand that few people these days like to spend tons of time in the kitchen, myself included. Be patient with yourself if you're new to cooking. Don't be afraid to make mistakes and experiment. Over time, things will get easier, and you'll get the hang of it. This is especially true when your heartburn and digestive issues start to fade. Cooking will simply become a part of your daily routine. You may even start to enjoy it!

# 15

# Recipes

One thing I've learned about cooking is that it's rare that I ever follow a recipe exactly as it's written. Sometimes I don't have all the spices or vegetables. No big deal. I'll just exclude them. Sometimes I'll want more or less of an ingredient as well. For example, I love garlic. Whenever I see a recipe that includes garlic, I almost always double, if not triple, it. And I rarely measure things out. To me, a teaspoon of salt means tilting the saltshaker for about three to four seconds (I have one that can flow more than sift). A tablespoon means a few more seconds than that. A half teaspoon of something means a few generous pinches.

You'll see that most of these recipes below contain amounts that are flexible. A little less or more of something is usually a matter of personal preference. Don't worry too much about precise amounts. The most important thing is to remember meal planning tip #5—have fun!

# Fermented Vegetables

# Easy-peasy Sauerkraut

**YouTube video demo: (http://bit.ly/1BvCcZG)**

**Ingredients**

- One medium head cabbage
- 1-2 Tbsp sea salt
- 1-2 Tbsp whey, optional
- 1-2 tsp caraway seeds, optional

**Directions**

1. Chop cabbage any way you want; thick or thin strips are fine. Hand chop or use a food processor, but don't blend up too fine.
2. Mix with salt in a large bowl.
3. Cover bowl and leave at room temperature for three to four hours or even longer. The salt will withdraw the water from the cabbage, making it very easy to pack into jars.
4. Cabbage should now be good and wet. Add whey and caraway seeds if using and mix with cabbage. Whey acts as a starter but it's not necessary. Caraway seeds add flavor. Take one handful of cabbage at a time and place in a wide mouth mason jar. Press and pack the cabbage into the jar with any kitchen instrument with a dull end. For years, I used the end of an eggbeater. Worked fine. These days I use a pastry maker that has a nice blunted end. The water should easily come out of the cabbage and start accumulating with every pressed handful. Continue pressing and packing until the cabbage is tightly packed and the water rises to one inch below the top of the jar.
5. Put lid on and leave at room temperature in a cool, dark place in your kitchen for three to seven days. It will ferment quicker in warmer weather.

6. Check it every day. Open the lid to relieve gases that build up. If the water starts to rise, let some out. If the cabbage starts to un-pack, pack it back down with your hands or a kitchen tool. If mold forms on the surface, don't freak out! Just remove it. This is a result of contact with air. Everything that is submerged in the brine is fine.
7. Taste the kraut after a few days. When it's pleasantly sour, transfer it to the fridge where it will continue to ferment and last for months and months.
8. Enjoy!

## Tips/Variations

1. You don't have to pre-salt the cabbage. It just means you'll be spending a little more time and muscle pounding the juices out of the cabbage if you don't.
2. Add other vegetables for different flavor and color combinations. Red cabbage, carrots, radishes, garlic, and onions are just a few suggestions. Personally, I love my sauerkraut plain. Experiment and find whatever works for you.
3. Double or triple the recipe for multiple jars. You can also use large crocks to make more at once, but I would recommend starting with smaller mason jars in case you don't like the initial results. As you gain experience and confidence, you can gravitate to larger fermenting vessels.
4. Whey acts as a starter culture by adding good bacteria but it's not necessary. To make whey, add a quart of good-quality yogurt to a cheesecloth-lined strainer set over a bowl for four to five hours. The yellowish liquid that drips out is whey. Transfer this to a jar in your fridge. It will last about six months. Tie the cheesecloth together and let it hang to let even more whey drip out. The yogurt will thicken further and you can add salt and herbs to it to make a delicious homemade cream cheese.

# Beginner's Kimchi

Kimchi is a spicy Korean sauerkraut. If spice aggravates your heartburn, you may have to wait before attempting this one. Still, I'm confident that you'll be able to include it after your symptoms start to fade.

My first forays into kimchi were fantastic failures. I could never get the spice and flavor right. My first few attempts were plain awful. Thanks to Sandor Katz in his book, *Wild Fermentation*, I learned a trick that I've used ever since. Hot sauce. This may not be the most traditional method, but it works beautifully. I've found I can consistently create the perfect amount of heat and spice that I like. I use two tablespoons of a medium hot sauce per one-quart mason jar. This suits my tastes perfectly, which is pretty spicy. Use more or less depending on how spicy you like it.

## Ingredients

- 1 Chinese cabbage (also called Napa cabbage)
- 2-4 cloves garlic, chopped
- 1-2 inches of fresh ginger root, grated or finely chopped
- 2-4 inches of daikon radish or 2-3 red radishes, sliced
- 1/2-1 bunch scallions, chopped
- 1-2 carrots, grated
- 1-2 Tbsp sea salt
- 2 Tbsp medium spicy hot sauce

## Directions

1. Chop cabbage as desired.
2. Mix all other ingredients except the hot sauce in a large bowl. Squeeze the vegetables in your hands until the juices start coming out. This is much easier than sauerkraut as the Chinese cabbage is less fibrous.
3. Thoroughly mix in the hot sauce.

4. Pack into mason jars until liquid rises to one inch below the top.
5. Leave at room temperature and check every day just like with sauerkraut.

## Tips/Variations

1. You can also soak the cabbage in a salty brine for a few hours or mix all the ingredients together and let them sit. This will also withdraw the water easily. Some say the former will add depth of flavor. I never do this, though.
2. Instead of hot sauce, the more traditional method is to add a dried red pepper powder. You can find authentic Korean versions in Asian markets. Make a paste by blending the ginger, garlic, and red pepper powder. Add to vegetables. Experiment with different amounts of spice to get the flavor you want.
3. If you're making kimchi for the first time, try different amounts of spice with each batch. After chopping and mixing all the vegetables together, put equal amounts into two or three separate bowls. Mix different amounts of spice in each bowl that you'll then pack into separate jars. Label each jar with the exact amounts of spice you've added. Whichever one you like best, write it down so you don't forget!

# Crunchy Dill Pickles

**YouTube video demo: (http://bit.ly/1CVDZ8q)**

Because pickles absorb water easily, they can easily turn to mush in the fermentation process. To avoid this, look for small, dark green, firm, and slightly under-ripe cucumbers. Trim off any stems. Check them every day especially in warmer weather. Move them to the fridge as soon as they turn sour and salty.

## Ingredients

- 3-4 small to medium pickling cucumbers (quartered, halved, or whole) per pint-sized jar
- One bunch dill
- 1-2 Tbsp sea salt
- 1-4 cloves garlic, optional
- 1-2 Tbsp pickling spices from your health food store, optional

## Directions

1. Place one clump dill and 1-2 cloves garlic at bottom of jar.
2. Pack pickles tightly in jar. Quartered and halved ones will fit easier than whole ones.
3. Add remaining garlic, pickling spices and another clump of dill and push gently into spaces between the cucumbers.
4. Add salt.
5. Cover with filtered water. Leave an inch between the top of the jar and the top of the water.
6. Cover lightly with lid and leave in a cool, dark place in your home.
7. Transfer to fridge after 2-4 days.

## Tips/Variations

1.  1. If you can't find a pre-prepared pickling spice in your health food store, you can make your own. Mix 1/4 to 1/2 tsp of each of the following spices:

- black peppercorns
- mustard seeds
- coriander seeds
- red pepper flakes
- allspice berries
- juniper berries
- whole cloves
- ground ginger

If you don't have one of the above, don't sweat it. Don't be afraid to experiment and add other spices too, like a cinnamon stick or other dried hot peppers.

# Fermented Beverages

# Beet Kvass

**YouTube video demo:** (http://bit.ly/1AYHmMK)

## Ingredients

- 2-3 medium beets, chopped into 1-inch cubes
- 2 Tbsp sea salt
- 1/4 cup whey, optional

## Directions

1. Add beets to a large 2-quart mason jar.
2. Add salt and whey.
3. Cover with filtered water. Leave an inch between the top of the jar and the top of the water.
4. Cover with lid and leave in a cool dark place in your home.
5. Transfer to fridge after 3-7 days.

## Tips/Variations

Beet kvass was never my favorite, but then I learned to add cabbage and onion, and now I absolutely love it. Chop about a cup or two of cabbage and a quarter to a half an onion. Place cabbage and onion on the bottom of the jar and then place beets firmly on top. Continue with steps 2-5.

# Ginger Ale

## Ingredients

- 3/4 cup fresh ginger, peeled and diced
- 1/4–1/2 cup fresh lime juice
- 2 tsp sea salt
- 1/4–1/2 cup rapadura, sucanat, or organic raw cane sugar
- 1/4 cup whey, optional
- 2 quarts filtered water

## Directions

1. Peel and chop ginger.
2. Add other ingredients to 2-quart glass jar and add filtered water.
3. Cover with filtered water. Leave an inch between the top of the jar and the top of the water.
4. Cover with lid and leave in a cool dark place in your home.
5. Transfer to fridge after 3-7 days.

## Tips/Variations

1. Don't buy pre-bottled lime juice! I did this once, and it completely ruined the batch. Bottled lime (and lemon) juices are often very concentrated and can make the taste way too limey.
2. Don't expect this to taste like the overly sweetened, chemical-laded store-bought stuff. Because this recipe is lacto-fermented, it will probably be stronger than most ginger ales you've tried in the past. If it's too strong, dilute it with some carbonated water. The carbonated water will also add some additional fizz.
3. Fizzing is a good sign that the fermentation is going well. Look for bubbling, which usually happens after 2-3 days. Be sure to taste it as you go. Your taste buds will tell you when it's ready.

# Kombucha

## Ingredients

- 1 kombucha mushroom ("mother")—you'll need to find a live culture from someone in your community or order one online in dehydrated form (www.culturesforhealth.com)
- 4 quarts filtered water
- 1 cup white organic sugar
- 4 organic black tea bags
- 1/2 cup kombucha from previous batch or from store

## Directions

1. Boil water.
2. Add sugar and stir to dissolve.
3. Remove from heat, add tea bags, and let steep until water cools to room temperature. Remove tea bags.
4. Add cooled liquid along with 1/2 cup kombucha to separate large glass container or bowl. Place kombucha mushroom on top.
5. Cover with a towel and secure with a rubber band to keep insects out. Place in a dark, cool corner of your kitchen.
6. Taste after 7 days. It shouldn't be sweet or taste like iced tea as the bacteria from the kombucha mother will convert the sugar and caffeine into beneficial substances. If it does taste sweet, continue to let it ferment and continue to taste it every day. It will ferment more quickly in warmer weather. When it's slightly sour and fizzy without being sweet, it's done. Transfer it to glass containers for storage in the fridge.

## Tips/Variations

7. When you have a cup or two left, repeat the above process. Your "mother" will have grown another! This will happen with every new batch. You can leave it as is or you can separate the two and give them away to friends. Peel them apart slowly and delicately, as they will bind to each other a bit.

8. The kombucha mothers can last for quite a long time. You'll know it's time to get another one when it starts to get a little funky looking or if your brew stops souring.

# The Three Basic Stocks

# Chicken Stock

**YouTube video demo:** (http://bit.ly/1zTB37E)

## Ingredients

- 1 whole chicken or chicken parts, cut up
- Vegetables, coarsely chopped—2-3 carrots, 2-3 stalks celery, 1 medium to large onion
- 1 – 2 Tbsp apple cider vinegar
- Chicken feet, optional

## Directions

1. Chop veggies and place in crockpot with chicken. Cover with water, add vinegar, and let sit for 30-60 minutes. The vinegar aids in leaching the minerals from the bones.
2. Turn crockpot to low and cook for 12-24 hours. That's it!
3. Strain broth from bones and veggies.
4. Store in fridge for up to 7 days. Freeze whatever you won't use within a week.

## Tips/Variations

1. Depending on the strength of your crockpot, you can remove the chicken after 3-5 hours and remove the meat from the bones. It should be well cooked and very tender. Reserve the meat for chicken salad or for a wonderful chicken soup. Return bones to water and continue simmering for 12-24 hours.
2. You can also use a stockpot on the stove top instead of a crockpot. For a less flavorful broth, simmer for 4-8 hours.
3. Adding fresh herbs at the end of the simmering imparts additional minerals and flavors. Parsley and thyme are two common additions.
4. You can also do the above with just chicken bones. Save your bones in your freezer until you have enough to make

a stock. Add in some chicken backs and necks for more depth.

5. When the stock cools, a layer of fat will form on the surface. Despite what every fat-phobic recipe on the internet says, don't skim it off! It will act as a seal and keep your stock fresher in the fridge for a longer period. When you do break the seal, you can either save the fat for use in other recipes (gravies, sautéing, etc.) or dissolve it back into the broth. Dissolving it back is a matter of personal preference. It will make your broth a little heavier. Perhaps wonderful for a cold winter night but not so much for other uses. You can also feed it to your dog who will love you for it!

# Fish Stock

Fish stock is my personal favorite. I use it for miso soup, chowders, cioppinos, and an assortment of Asian-style seafood soups. It's also the quickest to make, as the thin bones need less time to simmer. You'll need to find a good source of fish. Check with your local fish market or the seafood department at a health food store. They often throw away the parts for a stock and will sell them to you very cheaply. Non-oily white fish, like cod, halibut, striped bass, haddock, snapper, and hake, are best for fish stocks.

## Ingredients

- 1 whole fish from your local fish market, filleted, including head and tail fins but with gills and guts removed
- Vegetables, coarsely chopped—2-3 carrots, 2-3 stalks celery, 1 medium to large onion
- 1 cup dry white wine, optional
- Optional herbs and spices:
- 1-2 bay leaves
- 1-2 Tbsp black peppercorns
- A few sprigs thyme and/or rosemary

## Directions

1. Add all ingredients except optional spices to stock pot or crockpot. Cover with water.
2. Bring to a gentle boil and skim any foam that rises to surface; lower heat to a gentle simmer. The foam or scum won't hurt you, so the skimming isn't even necessary. I rarely skim it off myself. Some say it affects the taste, but many say it doesn't. I've never noticed the difference. Skimming the foam will, however, result in a clearer broth.
3. Add optional spices and simmer for 1-8 hours.
4. Strain broth in fine mesh colander or cheesecloth-lined colander.

5. Let cool and refrigerate and/or freeze.

**Tips/Variations**

1. Flatter fish like flounder and sole need shorter cooking times. An hour is usually fine.
2. For a more fragrant broth, you can sauté the veggies in butter first until they are soft and then add the fish carcass, wine, and water.
3. After cooling, it's best to discard the fat that forms on the surface as the delicate polyunsaturated fats in fish are more susceptible to heat.

# Beef Stock

**YouTube video demo:** (http://bit.ly/1zTB37E)

Beef stock is a little more time intensive as the thicker bones require more exposure to heat to withdraw their nutrients. Meatier bones also should be roasted, as they'll impart a deeper, richer flavor. It's not totally necessary though, and I often skip it.

**Ingredients**

- About four pounds bones including marrow bones, meaty bones, and knuckle bones.
- Vegetables, coarsely chopped—2-3 carrots, 2-3 stalks celery, 1 medium to large onion
- 1/4 cup red wine vinegar
- 1 cup full-bodied red wine like cabernet or zinfandel, optional
- 1-2 Tbsp peppercorns, optional
- 2 bay leaves, optional
- A few sprigs thyme, optional

**Directions**

1. Place non-meaty bones and vegetables in stockpot or crockpot, cover with water, and add vinegar. Let sit for one hour.
2. Roast meaty bones in oven set at 400 degrees til browned (not charred!) for 15-30 minutes. Add to crockpot. Deglaze the drippings from the roasting pan by adding water or red wine over high heat and scraping with a spatula. Add deglazed drippings to pot.
3. Bring to a boil, skim scum that rises to surface, and reduce heat to a very gentle simmer.
4. Add wine, peppercorns, bay leaves, and thyme.
5. Simmer for at least 12 hours but as long as 72 hours.

6. Remove the bones and strain broth in a fine mesh or cheesecloth-lined colander.
7. Cool and transfer to fridge or freezer.

## Tips/Variations

1. If you can't get a good variety of bones, that's OK. Any bones will do. Work with what you have and what you can get. All of them will still impart valuable minerals and nutrients. The great thing about broths is that you can always spice them up after the fact. Some folks even prefer blander broths for that reason. You can even exclude the veggies for all of the above broths as well.
2. You can roast the vegetables with the meaty bones as well.
3. Simmering should be *very* gentle. Never rapidly boil the bones, which can affect the flavor. A good indication of the right temperature is a few bubbles rising to the surface here and there.
4. As with the chicken stock, save the fat that congeals at the surface with cooling!

# Simple 3-Step Soups

Now let's take the above stocks and make some simple soups. Use these examples as a springboard for improvising your own creations. For each stock, I am including one soup using just the broth and one heartier example. Each will have variations so that you can experiment.

If you ever get stuck, just search for new ideas on Google! I do this all the time and still marvel that I can find anything I want at the tip of my fingertips. Recipe books are great and a treasure when you find a good one, but with the advent of the digital age, you barely even need them anymore.

# Chicken Stock-Based Soups

# Basic Chicken Soup – Broth Example

## Ingredients

- Vegetables of your choice—carrots, broccoli, mushrooms, greens, leeks, spinach, celery, onions, etc.
- Herbs of choice—parsley, cilantro, chives, basil, thyme, oregano, and rosemary work well
- Chicken, reserved from stock, or fresh chicken, cut into small strips or cubes
- Chicken stock
- Olive oil or butter
- Salt and pepper

## Directions

1. Sauté harder vegetables in butter and/or olive oil until soft.
2. Add stock and cook 10-15 minutes to amalgamate flavors. You can also just add the hard vegetables to the stock and cook everything together.
3. Add soft vegetables (greens), herbs, and chicken and simmer until chicken is cooked through.
4. Salt and pepper to taste.

## Tips/Variations

1. Substitute half of the chicken stock with coconut milk for a coconut-chicken soup. Adjust the amounts of each to your liking.
2. Add a little white wine, tomatoes, basil, and/or other Italians herbs like parsley, oregano, and thyme, and dried mushrooms for an Italian primavera-esque variation.
3. To make a simple egg drop soup, after Step 2, whisk a few eggs separately in a bowl. Scoop out a little stock and mix with arrowroot powder. Add back to broth and stir for a minute or two to thicken. Add eggs to broth in a slow and

steady stream, gently stirring. Top with green onions and chopped tomatoes. Flavor with a little miso paste or soy sauce.

# Potato Leek Soup – Hearty Example

Creamy root vegetable soups are a heartier variation that uses chicken stock. Though root vegetables are starchy, these soups are easily digested yet still filling and can be helpful in the grain-free stage if you're craving carbs.

## Ingredients

- 2-4 leeks, sliced thin
- 2-4 Tbsp butter
- 2 pounds cubed or chopped potatoes
- 1 quart chicken stock
- Salt and pepper
- Herbs of your choice—dill, parsley, thyme, and basil all work well alone or in combos. I like parsley and chives.

## Directions

1. Sauté leeks in butter until soft but not browned.
2. Add chicken stock and potatoes and cook about 30-40 minutes until potatoes are softened. Blend or mash. Adjust amount of stock you add for a thinner or thicker consistency.
3. Add herbs and soft vegetables. Season to taste.

Serve with pastured bacon bits, crème fraiche, or sour cream.

## Tips/Variations

1. Try this with sweet potatoes, butternut squash, carrots, or beets. Mix in other veggies. For example, butternut squash with tomatoes or zucchini or whatever floats your boat! Or maybe fruit. Pears and apples go well with carrots or beets, for example.
2. Add coconut milk with the herbs and vegetables in Step 3 for additional creaminess. You could also add some heavy cream here if you're not avoiding dairy. Raw cream is ideal but you will be heating it so this is the one place where

you can use some pasteurized cream from your health food store. Just make sure it's good quality.

3.  You can use the basic formula above with almost any vegetable, even non-root vegetables like asparagus, broccoli, or zucchini. Because they're less starchy, you'll need to puree the soup in batches at the end if you want a creamier texture. Adding coconut milk or cream will add thickness. But you can make them thin too. Just experiment and find what you like!

# Chicken Stock-Based Soups

# Basic Asian Fish Soup – Broth Example

Fish stock–based soups are my absolute favorite. There are infinite variations with different fish, shellfish, vegetables, herbs, and spices. For me, though, there is something magical about ginger, garlic, and either fish sauce or soy sauce. These pair well with almost any fish stock.

## Ingredients

- 1 quart fish stock
- Any seafood you like—shrimp, scallops, mussels, clams, and meaty white fish work well
- 1 inch piece of ginger, diced
- 1-4 cloves garlic, diced
- Any greens you like
- Soy sauce and/or fish sauce to taste

## Directions

1. Sauté ginger and garlic in sesame, coconut, or olive oil until soft.
2. Add fish stock, bring to a rolling boil, and cook 10-15 minutes to infuse broth with garlic and ginger.
3. Add greens and seafood and simmer until seafood is cooked, a few minutes.
4. Add soy sauce or fish sauce to taste.

## Tips/Variations

1. Add other veggies such as mushrooms, scallions, or string beans.
2. Many Asian soups are spicy. If spiciness does not aggravate your heartburn, you can add some chilies or hot sauce like sriracha for some kick and flavor.
3. Add rice noodles (after grain-free stage). Cook them separately and then add at the end.

4. Top with bean sprouts, herbs like mint or basil, and a squeeze of lemon or lime.

# Thai Seafood Coconut Curries – Hearty Example

## Ingredients

- 1-2 cans coconut milk and equal parts fish stock
- Seafood of your choice—any mild white fish, shrimp, squid, scallops, or crab, or a combo of any of them
- 1-2 cups of your favorite sliced vegetables—red pepper, peas, mushrooms, onions, string beans, etc.
- 1-2 Tbsp red, yellow, or green curry paste
- 1-2 Tbsp fish sauce
- Juice of lime and/or lemon
- Fresh Thai basil leaves. Regular basil is okay as well.
- 1 stalk lemongrass, optional

Note: Curry pastes are a mix of ginger, garlic, and other spices. Green is the spiciest. Red is the mildest. Yellow (also known as massaman) is the sweetest. You can frequently find them in the Asian section of health food stores or at a specialty Asian supermarket.

## Directions

1. Heat the coconut milk and stock until it comes to a boil. Turn heat down to medium, add curry paste, and stir to dissolve. Stir paste in slowly to taste. Use less for the spicier curries.
2. Add fish sauce, vegetables, and lemongrass. Cook 5–10 minutes or until veggies are tender and crisp, stirring occasionally.
3. Stir in seafood until cooked.
4. Add in basil in last few minutes.
5. Add in more fish sauce and lime or lemon to taste.

## Tips/Variations

1. Play around with the ratio of coconut milk to fish stock to get the consistency you like. I tend to add more coconut milk to give it a creamier texture.
2. In place of seafood and fish stock, substitute chicken and chicken stock for a Thai chicken curry, or beef and beef stock for a Thai beef curry.
3. Leave out the stocks entirely and just use coconut milk. You can pour this over a bed of rice after the grain-free stage.

# Beef Stock–Based Soups

# Faux Pho – Broth Example

Pho is a traditional Vietnamese soup with beef stock. This is my simple variation adapted from the more traditional version, which is a bit more time consuming. I've had both and was amazed how closely my simple version came to the more traditional one. Purists would surely disagree, but I'm not interested in being a purist. I'm interested in quick, simple, and delicious. This fulfills all three.

## Ingredients

- 1 quart beef broth
- Flank steak, sirloin, or London broil, sliced as thinly as possible
- 2-inch piece of ginger, diced
- Fish sauce
- Rice noodles, optional
- Spices:
- 3-4 whole star anise, whole cloves, whole cardamom pods, black peppercorns
- 1/2 tsp fennel seeds and coriander seeds
- Accompaniments
- Sriracha sauce, optional
- Hoisin sauce, optional
- Fresh mint, basil, and/or cilantro, handful each
- Bean sprouts, handful
- 1 lime wedge

## Directions

1. Put spices in a small mesh bag, tea bag, or any thin piece of cloth that you can tie up with the spices inside. Alternatively, you can just add them loosely to the broth and strain them out later.

2. Simmer beef stock with ginger and spices for 30–60 minutes. Keep lid on pot, otherwise the stock will evaporate.
3. Prepare rice noodles (leave out for grain-free stage) according to package directions and set aside.
4. Put rice noodles and thin beef strips in bowl. Pour hot broth over them. The heat will cook the beef.
5. Add fish sauce to taste.
6. Add sriracha and hoisin sauce to taste, optional.
7. Top with mint, basil, and/or cilantro; bean sprouts; and a squeeze of lime. You don't have to use all three herbs. I often just use one. Mint is my personal preference.

**Tips/Variations**

1. You can use beef broth in place of the fish broth in the Asian fish soup recipe above. Substitute some seared beef strips for fish. Use buckwheat noodles instead of rice noodles. Use soy sauce instead of fish sauce. Top with a little sesame oil and green onions. Serve with a side of kimchi. Create whatever variation you want from this variation!
2. If Pho is too foreign to you, stick with more familiar beef-broth soups. In the chicken soup recipe above, you can use beef broth in place of chicken broth for a simple beef vegetable soup.
3. French onion soup is another standard beef broth–based soup. I love this simple version by Jenny McGruther of Nourished Kitchen:
   http://nourishedkitchen.com/french-onion-soup/.
   Make sure to leave out the sourdough bread if you're using this while going grain-free.

# Quick and Easy Cabbage-Beef Stew – Hearty Example

Cookbooks will often have soups and stews grouped together. Stews are, well, stewier. They usually use tougher cuts of meat that require longer heating to break down, which is usually red meat like beef and lamb. Thus, they require a longer cooking time. But you can also use ground beef for a quicker stew. Cooking stews uses the same basic 3-step process as soups. In fact, it's more of a 2-step process as stews cook everything together so you won't often see step three.

## Ingredients

- 1-2 pounds ground beef
- 1 quart beef broth
- 1/2 cup red wine, optional
- 1 small to medium cabbage, cored and chopped
- 3-4 small red potatoes, quartered, optional
- 2-3 medium tomatoes or 1 can diced tomatoes
- 1 small jar tomato paste
- 1 medium onion
- 2-4 cloves garlic
- Italian seasonings—dried basil, thyme, and oregano
- Salt and pepper

## Directions

1. Sauté onions, garlic, and beef in olive oil, ghee, or other cooking fat until beef is browned.
2. Add everything else, stir, and cook on low heat until cabbage is cooked to desired consistency and potatoes are soft—about 30 minutes. Then season to taste. Make a large amount and use throughout the week.

## Tips/Variations

1. Use a crockpot instead. Simply add everything to the crockpot and cook on low for 4–8 hours.
2. I like to make a chicken stew with just chicken meat, some chicken stock, tomatoes, and tomato paste for thickening. You can do the same with seafood and fish stock.

# Salad Dressings and Mayo

The bad news is that it is nearly impossible to find a mayo or salad dressing without the quadruple bypass (corn, cottonseed, canola, soybean oil). Slightly healthier versions may use sunflower or safflower oil, but those are not much better. Refined vegetable oils aside, conventional salad dressings are a processed food nightmare full of sugar and chemicals.

The good news is that it is incredibly easy to make your own. Salads with a good protein will be helpful if you're a working person going through the grain-free stage. Homemade vinaigrettes and creamy dressings that use mayo as a base will help add some good healthy fats.

# Basic Vinaigrette

Vinaigrettes are simply an emulsion of oil and vinegar that is often mixed with other spices and seasonings. This basic vinaigrette uses mustard as a weak emulsifier.

## Ingredients

- 3/4 cup olive oil
- 1/4 cup balsamic vinegar
- 1 Tbsp organic Dijon mustard

## Directions

1. Combine vinegar and mustard in bowl.
2. Slowly drizzle in olive oil and whisk well.

## Tips/Variations

1. Make an herb vinaigrette by adding any chopped herbs you want.
2. For a different flavor, try other vinegars like apple cider, red wine, and rice vinegar.
3. Make a honey mustard vinaigrette by adding a tablespoon of honey to the basic vinaigrette. Use a white or red wine vinegar in place of balsamic.
4. Make a fruit vinaigrette by adding either fruit or the juice of the fruit. To make a raspberry vinaigrette, add fresh or thawed frozen raspberries to the basic formula and blend. To make an apple balsamic vinaigrette, add about a 1/4 cup apple cider to the basic formula and use apple cider vinegar instead of balsamic. Add some honey if it's not sweet enough. Add some chopped garlic and/or onion for more depth.
5. Add citrus. To make a lemon-lime or orange vinaigrette, squeeze the fresh juice to taste into the basic vinaigrette and mix. Add any herbs or spices you want. Try a different oil for different flavor combinations. Ideas: Lemon-

Sesame-Ginger, Orange-Thyme-Poppy seed, Cilantro-Lime-Walnut.

# Creamy Dressings

If you're like me, vinaigrettes are okay, but creamy dressings make salads a lot more filling and satisfying. Like most, I grew up with the store-bought versions and, to this day, my favorite salad dressing is Hidden Valley ranch. But I won't eat it anymore. Check out the label and you'll understand why.

Below are recipes for the three most common creamy dressings—blue cheese, Caesar, and ranch. Ranch almost always uses mayo as a base. Blue cheese often does as well though it's not completely necessary. The use of mayo will thicken these dressings a little once you put them in the fridge.

# Caesar

**YouTube video demo:** (http://bit.ly/1Ez1qnP)

## Ingredients

- 1 cup olive oil
- 2 egg yolks
- 1-2 cloves garlic, chopped
- 1-2 tsp Dijon mustard
- 1-2 Tbsp freshly squeezed lemon juice
- Salt and pepper to taste
- 2-3 anchovy fillets, optional

## Directions

1. Blend all ingredients except olive oil in food processor.
2. Add olive oil in a very slow and steady stream while continuing to blend.
3. Taste and add more mustard and lemon juice if needed. I will always start out with the smaller amounts above for this reason. Add salt and pepper to taste.

Note: Anchovies add a very fishy taste, which is a classic component of Caesar dressing. Some love it, some don't. Leave it out if need be. If you're not sure, add some anchovy fillets on the side of a Caesar salad first.

# Mayonnaise

**YouTube video demo:** (http://bit.ly/17BBBZ5)

## Ingredients

- 1 cup olive oil
- 1 whole egg
- 1 egg yolk
- 1-2 Tbsp lemon juice
- 1-2 tsp Dijon mustard
- Salt and pepper to taste
- 1 Tbsp whey, optional

## Directions

1. Blend all ingredients except olive oil in food processor.
2. In a very slow and steady stream, add the olive oil as the food processor is running. You can do this by hand as well but make sure to whisk vigorously. Adding olive oil in this manner will help thicken the mayo.
3. Leave at room temperature for 6–8 hours and transfer to fridge.
4. If adding whey, the mayo should keep in your fridge for several months. Without whey, it will keep for several weeks.

# Blue Cheese Dressing with Mayo

## Ingredients

- 4-6 ounces crumbled Blue Cheese
- 1 cup mayo or 1/2 cup mayo and 1/2 cup sour cream
- 1 Tbsp apple cider or wine vinegar
- 1 clove garlic, chopped or 1/2-1 teaspoon garlic powder
- 1 teaspoon Worcestershire sauce, optional
- Salt and pepper to taste

## Directions

Blend or whisk all ingredients together. Refrigerate.

# Blue Cheese Dressing Without Mayo

This is a simple version you can whip up in no time.

**Ingredients**

- 1/2 cup basic vinaigrette
- 2-4 ounces crumbled blue cheese, depending on how creamy you want it

**Directions**

1. 1. Mash blue cheese into vinaigrette until creamy. That's it!

# Ranch Dressing

## Ingredients

- 1 cup mayonnaise or 1/2 cup mayo and 1/2 cup sour cream.
- 1-2 Tbsp fresh parsley, minced
- 1-2 Tbsp fresh chives, minced
- 1-2 Tbsp fresh dill, minced
- 1-2 Tbsp scallions, chopped
- 1 clove garlic, chopped or 1/2–1 teaspoon garlic powder
- Salt and pepper to taste

## Directions

1. Combine all ingredients and let sit at room temp for an hour. Transfer to fridge.
2. Taste and adjust as necessary. More chives and scallions will add more of an onion flavor.
3. Dried herbs can be used, but fresh is always best.

# Grain-Free Breads

It's one thing to go without rice, cereals, and even pasta, but it's another to go without the soft, squishy, comforting goodness of bread. "But I loooooove bread!" says almost everyone when I recommend going grain-free. Brows wrinkle. Lips quiver. Shoulders slump. If that describes you, take some deep breaths and relax. Everything will be okay. I promise. Remember, the grain-free stage is only *temporary*. In the meantime, you can make some grain-free bread and other baked goods as a crutch.

There are two types of flour you can substitute for grain flours—coconut flour and nut flours. You can usually find them in your health food store, though it's not hard to make your own nut flour. Basically, just take some nuts and grind them up in a blender. It's really that simple.

Baking with alternative flours yields a thicker bread than store-bought versions. This is because there's no gluten! It may take some getting used, but I find most people enjoy heartier breads once they gravitate away from the highly processed ones. You may also have to play around with the ingredients. The amounts are not an exact science. I seem to get better results with coconut flour, but that's just me. To be honest, baking is not my strong suit. Below are two simple recipes to get you going, one using coconut flour and one using nut flour.

Finally, if you love to bake and/or just can't imagine going without your favorite baked goods, there are many great grain-free resources out there. Please see the <u>Heartburn Resourses Page</u> section for a few recommended options.

# Savory Coconut Flour Bread

## Ingredients

- 3/4 cup coconut flour
- 6 eggs
- 1/3–1/4 cup butter or ghee, melted
- 1 medium red onion, minced. Important: do not puree the onion as it will make the bread too soggy.
- 2 Tbsp honey
- 1/2 tsp sea salt

## Directions

1. Grease a bread loaf pan with butter, ghee, olive oil, or coconut oil.
2. Mix all of the above ingredients (except for onions) until there are no lumps and fill the loaf pan three-quarters full.
3. Bake in preheated oven at 350 degrees for about 40 minutes or until a knife is inserted into the middle and comes out clean.
4. Allow bread to cool before removing from pan. To remove, gently run a butter knife around the outside edges. Flip the pan over and it should come out in one piece.

# Almond Flour Bread

## Ingredients

- 3 cups almond flour
- 1/4 cup melted butter or coconut oil
- 4-5 eggs
- 1 tsp baking soda
- 1/2-1 tsp sea salt
- /2-1 tsp apple cider vinegar

## Directions

Same as coconut flour bread.

## Tips/Variations

1. To make banana bread, add 1-2 ripe bananas and a 1/4–1/2 cup of honey.
2. Add a 1/2–1 cup plain yogurt or crème fraiche for a more savory flavor.

# 16

## Grain-Free Meal Ideas

# Breakfast Ideas

## Eggs

Scramble 'em, poach 'em, hard-boil 'em, fry 'em, sunny side up 'em, frittata 'em, omelet 'em, etc. Whatever and however you like them. You can't go wrong with eggs for breakfast. Sauté with butter or coconut oil. Add cheese. Sides include organic/pastured bacon or sausage, salmon lox, and/or sautéed veggies—onions, peppers, zucchini, spinach, kale, etc. Whatever you like!
Here are just a few ideas:

- 2-3 poached eggs over a bed of spinach with avocado slices on the side.
- Scrambled eggs sautéed in butter with mushrooms and tomatoes, topped with cheddar cheese. Two bacons strips on the side.
- 2-3 sunny side up eggs over hash browns with a side of greens.
- 2-3 egg omelet with or without cheese of your choice and a side of sausage.
- 2-3 eggs over easy with a thick slice of toasted and buttered coconut or almond bread.

## Soups

It's funny how little variety there is for breakfast in America. Cereal or eggs about sums it up for the majority. Sometimes we have to think outside the box! Soup for breakfast may sound unusual, but it is a staple in many countries. Soups are a perfect morning meal as they are light yet filling and easy to digest. If eggs make you feel heavy or you're just not hungry for breakfast, consider soups. Prepared in advance, a simple reheat is all you need for those rushed AM hours.

See the ideas in the recipe section to get you started.

## Smoothies

Breakfast smoothies are perfect for those rushed morning hours. All you need is a good blender and three essential components: fruit, protein, and a healthy liquid.

1. Fruit. Add whatever you like! Blueberries, strawberries, raspberries, peaches, apples, bananas, oranges, pineapples, avocado, etc.

   Note: Avoid adding fruit juice, which is stripped of fiber and higher in sugar. If you're in a pinch, it's okay here and there but avoid the commercial varieties, which are usually non-organic, pasteurized, and contain added sugars and preservatives. You can also add a little raw honey if using more bitter fruits like apples and pears.

2. Protein. Nuts, nut butters, raw eggs from pastured chickens, and organic whole milk yogurt (unsweetened) are all excellent protein sources.

   Note: Protein powders are often processed at high temperatures and full of synthetic chemicals. I don't recommend them, but if you're going to use them, I'd recommend whey protein. Just be sure to choose a minimally processed product. And look for products that are protein concentrates, not protein isolates, which are more processed.

3. Healthy liquid. Raw whole milk or cream, kefir, almond milk, coconut milk, coconut water, and filtered water can all be used interchangeably. Use whatever you like!

You can also add vegetables. They are not essential but certainly a great complement to smoothies as well. Carrots and beets add a nice sweetness. Greens add in a powerful antioxidant punch as well as help detoxify the liver. Ginger is a common addition to smoothies and is also a potent anti-inflammatory.

Combine all ingredients in blender and blend until smooth. Experiment with different amounts and combinations and find what works for you.

Other ideas:

## Salads with Good Protein

Salads are also rarely thought of as a breakfast food, but they're perfectly acceptable. See the *Lunch Ideas* section.

## Sausage and Veggies

Turkey, beef, pork, or chicken sausages grilled or sautéed. Serve with onions and peppers over a bed of spinach or any greens of your choice.

## Full Fat Yogurt or Cottage Cheese

Top with almonds, walnuts, and/or fruit of your choice.

## Pancakes/Muffins with Nut Flour

Nut flours can be a nice substitute for grain-based flours, especially if you're missing your typical carby breakfast. They can also be a nice crutch in the grain-free stage. You can often find nut flours in the gluten-free sections of supermarkets. Warning though, they're not cheap. Make sure to incorporate good healthy fats like butter and coconut oil.

# Lunch Ideas

## Romaine Lettuce–Wrapped "Sandwiches"

I know it's hard to imagine a sandwich without bread, but lettuce wraps can make a nice substitute as you try to reduce starchy and refined carbohydrates and/or go grain-free. After your grain-free period ends, be it two weeks or longer, choose sprouted grain or sourdough bread, as they are easier for the body to digest. All of the following can be served as salads as well. And here's another great place you can add your homemade mayo!

Here are just a few simple ideas:

- BLT – bacon, lettuce (as wrap), tomatoes, red onion, homemade mayo
- Canned wild salmon or tuna, onion and red pepper, salt, pepper, homemade mayo
- Avocado, cream cheese (homemade if possible), cucumbers, diced shrimp (optional)
- Egg Salad – chopped hardboiled egg, onion, red pepper, salt, pepper, homemade mayo
- Chicken salad – chopped apple, celery, onion, red pepper, salt, pepper, homemade mayo
- Sliced strip steak with tomatoes, onions, cheddar cheese, horseradish sauce/mayo
- Turkey breast with avocado, cheddar, lettuce, tomato, onion, mayo or pesto mayo

## Salads

Always include a good protein—chicken, shrimp, salmon, steak, etc.—and use whatever veggies you like. The ideas below are just a few suggestions.

- Chef's salad – veggies of choice, protein of choice, hardboiled eggs, sliced tomatoes, thinly sliced red onions, mushrooms, olives, homemade ranch or blue cheese dressing
- Caesar salad – protein of choice, hardboiled eggs, sliced red onions, homemade Caesar dressing
- Triple A salad – arugula, avocado, and almonds with protein of choice and a vinaigrette dressing
- Garden salad – garden veggies, walnuts or almonds, dried cranberries, protein of choice, mozzarella cheese or homemade yogurt cream cheese, fresh basil, Italian vinaigrette dressing
- Spinach salad – spinach, any protein, goat cheese, walnuts, dried cranberries with a vinaigrette

## Soup in a Thermos

Heat up your leftover homemade soup in the morning before work and it'll still be piping hot at lunch. Side ideas: salad, fermented vegetables, raw cheese, nuts.

## Stew in a Thermos

Also ideal for heating in the morning and staying hot all day!

## Hardboiled Eggs

Sides: apple slices, carrot and celery sticks, almond butter, raw cheese, full fat cottage cheese, avocado, olives, pickles.

## Fruit and Veggie Plate

With cheese slices, nuts and healthy dips like hummus, almond butter, guacamole, pesto, ranch or blue cheese dressing, cream cheese with herbs, etc.

## Antipasto

This is the traditional first course in Italian meals but can easily be a meal on its own. Includes cured meats like pepperoni and salami, sardines and anchovies, artichoke hearts, olives, marinated mushrooms, roasted red peppers, and a variety of cheeses. Mix and match for a great snack too.

## Leftover Dinner!

Slices of last night's beef roast, leftover chili, extra chicken cubed or diced, etc. Serve with veggies, a side salad, cheese slices, and/or fruit.

# Dinner Ideas

## Simple Baked Salmon

Top with a lemon-butter sauce with green veggies of choice. Or use whatever seafood you like—sole, cod, haddock, trout, grouper, snapper, swordfish, or scallops all work well.

## Baked Chicken Drumsticks

Rub with Italian herbs and seasonings, serve with green beans and roasted sweet potatoes or roasted turnips.

## Broiled Lamb Chops

Brush with olive oil, salt, and pepper and broil three to four minutes per side. Serve with kimchi, asparagus, Brussels sprouts, or green beans.

## Honey Mustard Pork Chops

Mix honey, mustard, olive oil, salt, and pepper. Brush chops with sauce and broil five to seven minutes per side until tender and browned. Serve with sauerkraut.

## Quick and Easy Sautéed Steak

Sauté steak with fish sauce and crème fraiche to taste. Serve with kimchi, spinach, kale, or side salad, and roasted sweet potato fries.

## Bacon Wrapped Sea Scallops

Cut bacon strips in half and wrap around scallops. Secure with a toothpick through middle of scallop. Broil about four to five inches from heat and about three to five minutes per side or until bacon is crisp. Dipping sauce idea—mayo with lime, chopped cilantro, and sriracha hot sauce to taste.

## Ground Pork or Beef Cabbage Roll Ups

Sauté onions, garlic, ginger, and chili peppers (optional) in sesame or coconut oil. Add ground meat and cook through. Add soy sauce to taste. Scoop into steamed cabbage leaves and roll. Serve with sauerkraut or kimchi.

## Soups!

See Recipes Section

## Chilis and Stews

Like soups, these are also great to cook in bulk and store for use later in the week. Slow cookers are ideal for both and cut down on cooking time.

## Stir Fries

Make a cauliflower or cabbage "rice" by blending either one in food processor until it resembles rice. Sauté until tender, about five to ten minutes. Add other veggies and protein.

Classic combos:

Thai – coconut milk, fish sauce, chilies, basil, peanuts

Japanese – sesame oil, ginger, garlic, soy sauce

Chinese – soy sauce, rice wine, arrowroot powder (to thicken), and a little coconut sugar or rapadura sugar

Mexican – homemade taco seasoning (chili powder, paprika, cumin, garlic powder, onion powder, oregano, salt, pepper) with chopped lettuce, salsa, sour cream, avocado, and cheese on the side

## Zucchini "Pasta"

Using a vegetable peeler (use julienne peeler for thinner strips), slice two or three zucchini in long strips that resemble pasta noodles. Either sauté zucchini pasta in olive oil or butter for a few minutes until soft or boil in water for about a minute. Add any sauce (marinara, pesto, carbonara, scampi, primavera, butter with herbs and garlic, etc.) with any vegetable and protein you want.

# Healthy Snack Ideas

## The Sugar Buster

This will be very helpful if you experience sugar cravings during the initial phases. Mix together approximately equal parts nut butter and coconut oil. Add raw honey to taste. Experiment with the quantities to find what works for you. Store in a glass jar and keep near you at all times. Use as needed when cravings hit.

## Yogurt

Plain and FULL FAT! Optional: add fruit and/or nuts.

## Cheese (Preferably Raw) with Fruit or Veggies

Havarti with apple slices. Cheddar with carrot sticks. Goat cheese with grapes or strawberries.

## Hardboiled Eggs

With sea salt. Optional: w/cucumber slices, avocado.

## Nuts

Raw and preferably soaked overnight (with a little sea salt) and dried.

## Nut Butters

Good quality almond, cashew, peanut, or walnut butters. With any raw veggies—celery, carrots, etc. Apple slices work great too.

## Hummus and Veggies

## Trail Mix

Careful on the ones with a lot of chocolate and dried fruit.

## Dill Pickles (preferably homemade)

Optional: with cheddar cheese (it really works!)

## Avocado

Plain or with a squeeze of lemon or lime and sea salt. Optional: spread on sprouted grain bread with cuke or tomato slices.

## Smoothies

See "Smoothies" above in "Breakfast Ideas".

## Glass of Raw Milk (my personal favorite)

## Meats

Possibilities: leftover chicken or turkey, a few slices of good quality lunch meat (with a few slices of cheese), good quality beef or turkey jerky (try to find low sugar varieties), salmon jerky.

## Kombucha

A great sugar cravings buster! Sip at night or whenever cravings hit.

## Coconut Oil (spoonful)

Optional (though highly recommended): with a spoonful of the nut butter of your choice.

## Canned Salmon and Tuna

With good homemade mayo and chopped up veggies—onions, peppers, celery, etc. Optional: roll in a nice big piece of lettuce such as romaine for a makeshift wrap—great for lunch too.

## Lox and Cream Cheese

With veggies of your choice.

## Sardines or Anchovies

Not everyone's cup of tea but some love them (myself included).

## Kielbasa or Pepperoni Slices

With a pickle or two.

## Kale Chips

Remove leaves from stems and tear into small pieces. Drizzle in olive oil and sea salt and mix until lightly coated. Bake at 350 degrees until edges are brown but not burnt, for 10-15 minutes. Deelish!

# 17

# Grain-Free Meal Plans

As you'll see, these meal plans are very basic. Their purpose is just to give you some structure for creating a meal plan without it being overwhelming and overly time consuming. As such, they only include lunches and dinners and exclude the weekends. This will keep planning very simple. Breakfasts are very easy for most people as eggs, oatmeal (post grain-free stage), leftover soups, and smoothies can all be whipped up in a matter of minutes. And weekends are often difficult to plan for as travel plans and social situations are more likely. Use leftovers from the week if you can and don't stress the weekends. You also might be prepping some meals for the coming week that you can use for meals as well.

Here's how I do things. Start with dinners. Think of two to three dinners that you can cook in bulk and use as leftovers for lunch. For example, leftover meats can be used for salads. Soups can be warmed up in the morning and put in a thermos. Leftover chicken or fish can be diced and mixed with some mayo and veggies. Obviously, this will be a little more challenging if you're cooking for a family as opposed to just yourself. But you'll be so thankful later in the week when a simple reheat is all you need.

Next, plan your lunches. Since you've already planned some of them from dinner leftovers, this means you'll usually only need to come up with a few. And keep it simple. So for example, a fruit and vegetable plate with some cheese, some hardboiled eggs with cucumbers and avocado slices, or some canned tuna or salmon over a salad or as a romaine lettuce-wrapped sandwich.

Next, sketch out your week but don't be too regimented about it. Just have an idea of how things will go. Have quick and versatile ingredients on hand for those nights when you get home later than expected.

Finally, try to find one day of the week, more than likely the weekend, where you spend some time preparing things for the week.

And really that's it! So when you look at my meal plans, you'll notice it mostly revolves around planning just three or four meals each week. If you want to cook more, by all means go for it. But this sure beats making 21 different meals from scratch, doesn't it?

# Sample Grain-Free Weekly Meal Plan #1

## Weekly Dinners:

Potato leek soup
Chicken drumsticks or wings with side blue cheese dressing
Steak

## Weekly Lunches from Dinner Leftovers:

Potato leek soup
Steak salad/slices
Chicken drumsticks/wings

## Weekend Planning and Prep:

Make chicken stock for soup
Make blue cheese dressing
Hard-boil a dozen or so eggs for salads

## Monday

Lunch - Garden salad with hardboiled eggs and blue cheese dressing
Dinner - Grilled/sautéed steak with mushrooms and onions, roasted sweet potatoes, greens

## Tuesday

Lunch - Leftover steak slices with cheese slices and side salad
Dinner - Potato leek soup

## Wednesday

Lunch - Caesar salad with leftover steak slices
Dinner - Chicken drumsticks/wings with blue cheese dressing, green veggies

## Thursday

Lunch - Leftover chicken drumsticks/wings and blue cheese dressing with carrot and celery sticks
Dinner - Potato leek soup

## Friday

Lunch - Caesar salad with leftover steak slices or any protein of choice
Dinner - Potato leek soup

# Sample Grain-Free Weekly Meal Plan #2

## Weekly Dinners:

Whole roast chicken
Baked salmon
Faux pho

## Weekly Lunches from Dinner Leftovers:

Chicken Caesar salad
Faux pho

## Weekend Planning and Prep:

Make beef stock for pho
Make Caesar dressing
Hard boil eggs

## Monday

Lunch - Hardboiled eggs, pickles, side salad
Dinner - Roast chicken, side fermented vegetable, sweet potatoes

## Tuesday

Lunch - Chicken Caesar salad with chicken leftovers
Dinner - Baked salmon, green vegetable

## Wednesday

Lunch - Salmon salad from leftover salmon over bed of greens
with hardboiled egg slices
Dinner - Faux pho, kimchi

## Thursday

Lunch - Pho in a thermos, pack accompaniments on the side
Dinner - Eat out/order out or quick and easy eggs with side veggies

## Friday

Lunch - Caesar salad with chicken leftovers
Dinner - Faux pho, kimchi

# Final Thoughts and THANK-YOU

I hope the ideas in this book were beneficial and opened up some new ways of dealing with your heartburn. I want to share just a few final thoughts to put things in perspective.

## 1. Real food is a lifelong journey.

Obviously, what I've laid out in this book is about a lot more than just heartburn. It's also about real food. And if you're new to real food, it can take some time to reorient around it. It may mean driving a little further to the good quality supermarket, budgeting a little more money, and of course, cooking more.

Know that *almost everyone* is on this journey, as well. And that includes me. Like most Americans, I grew up on processed food. It wasn't until my mid-20s that I started cooking for myself and it wasn't until my 30s that I started incorporating the ideas in this book.

*I'm always learning.* You will make things that will WOW you. And you will make things that will make you pick up the phone and order out. That's just part of it.

Don't be afraid to learn from your mistakes.

## 2. Let go of perfectionism

Yes, it is good to be as strict as possible in the grain-free stage. Yes, you may uncover a gluten sensitivity. Yes, it is good to source more real food and make better choices. But over the long term, being perfect is not possible. Don't stress it when you find yourself in situations where there is nothing you can do— airports, sporting arenas, or perhaps a holiday trip to a relative.

There is something to be said for the 80-20 rule; that is, if you eat real food 80% of the time, you can probably get away with eating not-so-real food 20% of the time.

## 3. Be patient

Again, how quickly things resolve depends on a number of factors. Chronic cases may take more time. Thirty years of GERD is unlikely to disappear overnight. Be patient.

## 4. If you need more help

If you feel you need more guidance and support, check out my online digestive wellness course, Fearless Digestion. The course contains eight digestive health modules that you progress through at your own pace. Module topics include many of the topics discussed here (healthy fats, grains, fermented foods, bone broths, etc.) but in a bit more depth. There are additional recipes, handouts, and cooking videos and a support forum for class members. Course details are over at www.fearlessdigestion.com

## 5. Thank you!

Thank you so much for taking the time to read my book. I genuinely hope it will change your life.

If you have questions or comments, feel free to contact me through the contact page of my website, www.fearlesseating.net. I'd love to hear from you. And I especially love testimonials! It makes me feel good when you feel good. So don't hesitate to let me know how this book has helped you.

And let's stay in touch!

Please join me on Facebook: www.facebook.com/FearlessEating

On Google +: plus.google.com/+FearlesseatingNetPlus

And on Pinterest: pinterest.com/fearlesseating

Thank you again and I wish you all the best on your journey with real food and a heartburn-free life!

Warmly,

Craig

# One Small Request

Thanks so much for reading my book. I genuinely hope you've found it helpful. If so, I would greatly appreciate it if you would take a moment to write a brief review on Amazon. Reviews mean a great deal to me and will help others suffering with heartburn to find this book, so that they too can find relief from heartburn suffering. Thank you so much!

# Get More!

Please visit my website at www.fearlesseating.net and subscribe to my mailing list so that we can keep in touch. I plan to write many books in the future and will notify you of their releases and promotional discounts. No spam, you have my word! You'll also get free recipes, digestive health tips, and more great info to support you on your heartburn-free journey!

# References

## Chapter 1

1. National Institute of Diabetes and Digestive and Kidney Diseases, U.S. Dept of Health and Human Services. Digestive Diseases Statistics for the United States. N.p., 10 May 2012. Web. 7 March 2013. <http://digestive.niddk.nih.gov/statistics/statistics.aspx>.

2. Ibid.

## Chapter 3

1. Wright, Jonathan V., and Lane Lenard. Why Stomach Acid Is Good for You: Natural Relief from Heartburn, Indigestion, Reflux, and GERD. New York: M. Evans, 2001. 20 p.

2. Ibid.

3. Lovat, L. B. "Age Related Changes in Gut Physiology and Nutritional Status." Gut 38.3 (1996): 306-09. Web. 9 March 2013.

4. Konturek P.C., T. Brzozowski , S.J. Konturek. "Stress and the gut: pathophysiology, clinical consequences, diagnostic approach and treatment options." Journal of Physiology and Pharmacology 62.6 (2011): 591-99. Web. 9 March 2013.

5. Mönnikes H., J.J. Tebbe, M. Hildebrandt, P. Arck, E. Osmanoglou, M. Rose, B. Klapp, B. Wiedenmann, I. Heymann-Mönnikes. "Role of stress in functional gastrointestinal disorders. Evidence for stress-induced alterations in gastrointestinal motility and sensitivity." Digestive Diseases 19.3 (2001): 201-11. Web. 10 March 2013.

6. Kresser, Chris. "The Hidden Causes of Heartburn and GERD." Chris Kresser L.Ac: Medicine for the 21st Century.

N.p., 01 Apr. 2010. Web. 7 March 2012. chriskresser.com/the-hidden-causes-of-heartburn-and-gerd

## Chapter 4

1. Zaki M, P.E. Coudron, R.W. McCuen, L. Harrington, S. Chu, M.L. Schubert. "H. pylori acutely inhibits gastric secretion by activating CGRP sensory neurons coupled to stimulation of somatostatin and inhibition of histamine secretion." American Journal of Physiology. Gastrointestinal and Liver Physiology 304.8 (2013): G715-22. Web 3 April 2013.

2. Gershon, Michael D. The Second Brain. New York: HarperCollins World, 1999. 110 p.

3. Penagini, R, M. Mangano, and P.A. Bianchi. "Effect of increasing the fat content but not the energy load of a meal on gastro-oesophageal reflux and lower oesophageal sphincter motor function." Gut 42 (1998): 330-33. Web. 6 April 2013.

## Chapter 6

1. Siri-Tarion Patty, Qi Sun, Frank B. Hu and Ronald M. Krauss. "Meta-analysis of Prospective Cohort Studies Evaluating the Association of Saturated Fat with Cardiovascular Disease". The American Journal of Clinical Nutrition. 99.3 (2010): 535-546. Web. 6 May 2013.

2. Volk M.G. "An examination of the evidence supporting the association of dietary cholesterol and saturated fats with serum cholesterol and development of coronary heart disease." Alternative Medicine Review. 12.3 (2007):228-45. Web. 6 May 2013.

3. Jones PJ. "Dietary cholesterol and the risk of cardiovascular disease in patients: a review of the Harvard Egg Study and other data." International Journal of Clinical Practice 163.1-8. (2009): 28-36. Web. 6 May 2013.

## Chapter 7

1. Fallon, Sally, and Mary G. Enig PhD. "Be Kind to Your Grains." Weston A Price Foundation. N.p., 01 January 2000. Web. 19 May 2013. http://www.westonaprice.org/food-features/be-kind-to-your-grains

2. Ibid.

## Chapter 8

1. Yang WH, M.A. Drouin, M. Herbert, Y. Mao, J. Karsh. "The monosodium glutamate symptom complex: assessment in a double-blind, placebo-controlled, randomized study." Journal of Allergy and Clinical Immunology 99.6 Pt 1 (1997): 757-62. Web. 13 May 2013.

2. "CFR - Code of Federal Regulations Title 21." US Food and Drug Administration. N.p., 01 April 2012. Web. 14 May 2013. http://www.accessdata.fda.gov/scripts/cdrh/cfdocs/cfcfr/cfrsearch.cfm?fr=501.22.

3. "What Is MSG?" http://www.truthinlabeling.org : The Truth, the Whole Truth and Nothing but the Truth about MSG. N.p., n.d. Web. 21 May 2013. http://www.truthinlabeling.org/HowIsItManufactured.html.

4. Wright, Jonathan V., and Lane Lenard. Why Stomach Acid Is Good for You: Natural Relief from Heartburn, Indigestion, Reflux, and GERD. New York: M. Evans, 2001. p. 60-66, 72-73.

5. Targownik LE, L.M. Lix, C.J. Metge, H.J. Prior, S. Leung, W.D. Leslie. "Use of proton pump inhibitors and risk of osteoporosis-related fractures." Canadian Medical Association Journal. 179.4 (2008): 319-26. Web. 23 May 2013.

6. Yang YX, J.D. Lewis, S. Epstein, D.C. Metz. "Long-term proton pump inhibitor therapy and risk of hip fracture." Journal of the American Medical Association. 296.4 (2006): 2947-53. Web. 23 May 2013.

7. "Debunking the Myths." National Osteoporosis Foundation. N.p., n.d. Web. 24 May 2013. http://www.nof.org/articles/4.

8. "News & Events. FDA News Release. FDA: Possible Fracture Risk with High Dose, Long-term Use of Proton Pump Inhibitors." US Food and Drug Administration. US Dept. of Health and Human Services. 23 April 2013. Web. 26 May 2013. http://www.fda.gov/NewsEvents/Newsroom/PressAnnouncements/ucm213377.htm .

## Chapter 9

1. Langer, Adam J., Tracy Ayers, Julian Grass, Michael Lynch, Frederick J. Angulo, and Barbara E. Mahon. "Nonpasteurized Dairy Products, Disease Outbreaks, and State Laws – United States, 1993-2006." Emerging Infectious Diseases 18.3 (2012): 385-91. Web. 27 May 2013. http://wwwnc.cdc.gov/eid/article/18/3/pdfs/11-1370.pdf

2. "Food Safety for Moms-to-Be Power Point Presentation." US Food and Drug Administration. US Dept. of Health and Human Services. 16 April 2013. Web. 20 May 2013. http://www.fda.gov/Food/ResourcesForYou/HealthEducators/ucm095399.htm.

3. Mercola, Joseph. "The War Over Raw Milk Heats Up." Mercola.com. N.p., 14 August 2010. Web. 2 June 2013. http://articles.mercola.com/sites/articles/archive/2010/08/14/the-war-over-raw-milk-heats-up.aspx

4. Satchell, Michael, Steven J. Hedges, and Linda Kulman. "The Next Bad Beef Scandal?" US News. 24 August 1997. U.S.News & World Report. Web. 25 May 2013. http://www.usnews.com/usnews/news/articles/970901/archive_007713.htm.

5. McAfee, Mark. "The 15 Things That Milk Pasteurization Kills." A Campaign for Real Milk. 25 December 2012. Web. 25 May 2013 http://www.realmilk.com/commentary/15-things-that-milk-pasteurization-kills/.

6. Phelan, Benjamin. "The Most Spectacular Mutation in Human History." Slate Magazine. N.p., 23 October 2012. Web. 23 May 2013.
http://www.slate.com/articles/health_and_science/human_ev olution/2012/10/evolution_of_lactose_tolerance_why_do_hu mans_keep_drinking_milk.html.

## Chapter 10

1. Duggan, Tara. "Cultivating Their Fascination with Fermentation." SFGate. N.p., 7 June 2009. Web. 14 May 2013.
http://www.sfgate.com/food/article/Cultivating-their-fascination-with-fermentation-3295948.php#page-1

## Chapter 11

1. Thomas, Cowan. "Ask the Doctor: GERD." Weston A Price Foundation. N.p., 23 March 2003. Web 04 June 2013.
http://www.westonaprice.org/Ask-the-Doctor/

2. Hu T., K.T. Mills, L. Yao, K. Demanelis, M. Eloustaz, WS Yancy Jr., T.N. Kelly, J. He, L.A. Bazzano. "Effects of low-carbohydrate diets versus low-fat diets on metabolic risk factors: a meta-analysis of randomized controlled clinical trials." American Journal of Epidemiology. 176 Suppl 7 (2012):S44-54. Web. 10 May 2013

3. Brehm BJ, R.J. Seeley, S.R. Daniels, D.A. D'Alessio. "A randomized trial comparing a very low carbohydrate diet and a calorie-restricted low fat diet on body weight and cardiovascular risk factors in healthy women." Journal of Clinical Epidemiology and Metabolism. 88.4 (2003):1617-23. Web. 10 May 2013

4. Krebs Nancy F., Dexiang Gao, Jane Gralla, Juliet S. Collins, and Susan L. Johnson. "Efficacy and Safety of a High Protein, Low Carbohydrate Diet for Weight Loss in Severely Obese Adolescents." Journal of Pediatrics 157.2 (2010):252-258. Web. 10 May 2013

5. Samaha Frederick F., Nayyar Iqbal, Prakash Seshadri, Kathryn L. Chicano, Denise A. Daily, Joyce McGrory, Terrence Williams, Monica Williams, Edward J. Gracely, and Linda Stern. "A Low-Carbohydrate as Compared with a Low-Fat Diet in Severe Obesity." The New England Journal of Medicine. 348(2003):2074-2081. Web. May 10 2013

6. Davis, William. Wheat Belly: Lose the Wheat, Lose the Weight, and Find Your Path Back to Health. Emmaus, Penn.: Rodale, 2011. p. 14, 18, 25.

7. National Institute of Diabetes and Digestive and Kidney Diseases, U.S. Dept of Health and Human Services. Celiac Disease. N.p., 27 January 2012. Web. 25 May 2013. http://digestive.niddk.nih.gov/ddiseases/pubs/celiac/

## Chapter 12

1. Fallon, Sally, and Mary G. Enig. Nourishing Traditions: The Cookbook That Challenges Politically Correct Nutrition and the Diet Dictocrats. Washington, DC: NewTrends Pub., 2001. 610 p.

2. Daniels, Kaayla. "Why Broth Is Beautiful: Essential Roles for Proline, Glycine and Gelatin." Weston A Price Foundation. 18 June 2003. Web. 17 May 2013. http://www.westonaprice.org/food-features/why-broth-is-beautiful

3. Ibid.

4. Ibid.

5. Backing, Christopher. "Gelatin Treats Ulcer." Medical News Today. MediLexicon, Intl., 22 August 2006. Web. 17 May 2013. http://www.medicalnewstoday.com/releases/50126.php

6. Yamadera, W., K. Inagawa, S. Chiba, M. Banna, M. Takahashi, and K. Nakayama. "Glycine ingestion improves subjective sleep quality in human volunteers, correlating with

polysomnographic changes." Sleep and Biological Rhythms, 5.2 (2007)126–131. Web. 8 April 2013.

7. Lesbros-Pantoflickova D , I. Corthésy-Theulaz, A.L. Blum. "Helicobacter pylori and Probiotics." The Journal of Nutrition 137.3 (2007): 812S-818S. Web. 14 April 2013.

8. Mercola, Joseph. "This Food Contains 100 Times More Probiotics Than A Supplement." Mercola.com. 12 May 2010. Web 20 May 2013 http://articles.mercola.com/sites/articles/archive/2012/05/12/dr-campbell-mcbride-on-gaps.aspx

9. Crew, JR. "The Milk Cure: Real Milk Cures Many Diseases." A Campaign for Real Milk. N.p., 01 January 2000. 30 May 2013 http://www.realmilk.com/health/milk-cure/.

10. Beals, Ted. "Lactose Intolerance Survey." A Campaign for Real Milk. N.p., 17 December 2012. 31 May 2013 http://www.realmilk.com/health/lactose-intolerance-survey/

## Chapter 13

1. Wright, Jonathan V., and Lane Lenard. Why Stomach Acid Is Good for You: Natural Relief from Heartburn, Indigestion, Reflux, and GERD. New York: M. Evans, 2001. 138 p.

2. Reimer, Christina, Bo Søndergaard, Linda Hilsted, and Peter Bytzer. "Proton-Pump Inhibitor Therapy Induces Acid-Related Symptoms in Healthy Volunteers After Withdrawal of Therapy." Gastroenterology 137.1 (2009): 80-87.e1. Web. 15 June 2013

3. Campbell-McBride, Natasha. Gut and Psychology Syndrome: Natural Treatment for Autism, Dyspraxia, ADD, Dyslexia, ADHD, Depression, Schizophrenia. Cambridge, U.K.: Medinform Pub., 2010. p. 278-279.

4. Stumpf W.E. "Vitamin D and the Digestive System." European Journal of Drug Metabolism and Pharmacokinetics. 33.2 (2008): 85-100. Web. 29 April 2013

# About the Author

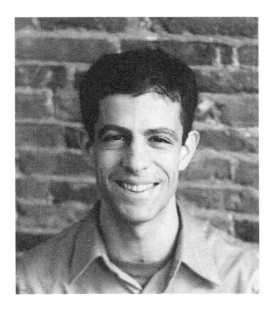

Hi there! My name is Craig Fear.

I'm a certified Nutritional Therapy Practitioner (NTP), and my practice, Pioneer Valley Nutritional Therapy, is located in Northampton, Massachusetts.

I also have a degree in biology from the University of Mary Washington, but my interest in nutrition didn't take hold until many years after I graduated. I had to explore life a little first before I found what I really wanted to do. I won't bore with you the details, but here's the ultra-short version of how I came to write this book:

My first gig out of college was a soul-crushing job at a pharmaceutical company in Rockville, MD. My life had become a scene out of the movie *Office Space*, the 90s classic about the drudgery of working a job you hate. If you've seen the movie, I worked in a place *exactly* like Initech. I hated it from the moment I started, and it ignited a burning desire in me to drive far, far away. So I did.

After a year, I quit, saved up some money, and drove west until I couldn't drive any farther, literally. I wound up in Homer, Alaska, a magical little town they call "the end of the road." I stayed for two years and met some wonderfully fascinating, creative, and inspiring people—fishermen, farmers, artists, homesteaders, musicians, mystics, and more.

Living in Homer kick-started a journey of self-discovery that led to travels to Thailand, India, and Burma. I became interested in eastern spirituality and began to practice yoga and meditation.

I also became a vegetarian for seven years. I did this not only for ethical and spiritual reasons but for health reasons as well. But something interesting happened over the course of those seven years. I started to develop chronic digestive issues. Though I experienced heartburn on occasion, my bigger problem was chronic bloating. I wasn't breaking down and absorbing the nutrients in my food efficiently, and I developed chronic fatigue as well.

As I learned later, my symptoms were very closely related to heartburn. Turns out, the diet I was eating was almost exactly the same one that causes the overwhelming majority of heartburn cases.

You may be thinking, "So the problem was being a vegetarian?" Not exactly. There's a lot more to it than that. I hadn't learned enough about nutrition at that point in my life to make better choices as a vegetarian.

Eventually, I gave up being a vegetarian and after reading this book, if you're also a vegetarian, you may too. Or not. That's not what this book is about.

But it is about diet and nutrition more than you might think. As you'll see, simple dietary changes are often all it takes to stop heartburn and its many related digestive symptoms.

I am confident that the ideas in this book will help you like they helped me. Who knows, it may even inspire you to become a Nutritional Therapist! OK, probably not, but that's what happened to me. I was so inspired by my own health transformation that I knew I had to help others as well. I completed my training as a Nutritional Therapist in the spring of 2008 and moved to western Massachusetts that fall to start my practice, where I continue to see clients in person and over the phone.

Though I see clients around a variety of health issues, my favorite clients are those with chronic heartburn. Why? Because it's so easy to turn around! And that's why I wrote this book.

Here are a few other things about me: I love to hike, play my guitar, travel, practice vipassana meditation when I can, root for my beloved New York Giants (I'm from New York), read about nutrition, and write about nutrition on my blog, *Fearless Eating*. I also love coffee and am only mildly addicted to it.

It's my sincere hope that this book will help you like it helped me.

Ready to start on a journey towards a heartburn-free life?

Let's do it.

Made in the USA
Monee, IL
11 January 2021

57265170R00121